FAST FACTS

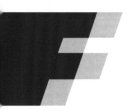

Indispensable

Guides to

Clinical

Practice

Hy[

Paul Durrington

Professor of Medicine, University of
Manchester, Department of Medicine,
Manchester Royal Infirmary, UK

Allan Sniderman

Edwards Professor of Cardiology
and Professor of Medicine,
McGill University, Montreal, Canada

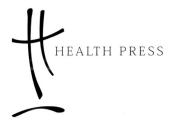

HEALTH PRESS

Oxford

Fast Facts – Hyperlipidaemia
First published 2000

Text © 2000 Paul Durrington, Allan Sniderman
© in this edition Health Press 2000
Health Press Limited, Elizabeth House, Queen Street, Abingdon,
Oxford OX14 3JR, UK
Tel: +44 (0)1235 523233
Fax: +44 (0)1235 523238

Fast Facts is a trade mark of Health Press Limited.

The authors are indebted to Caroline Price for her expert preparation of
the original manuscript and to the University of Manchester Department
of Medical Illustration, UK, for many of the figures. We also gratefully
acknowledge the great support of colleagues, particularly Paul Miller.
This book is dedicated to our wives.

A CIP catalogue record for this title is available from the British Library.

ISBN 1-899541-48-9

Durrington, P (Paul)
Fast Facts – Hyperlipidaemia/
Paul Durrington, Allan Sniderman

Illustrated by MeDee Art, London, UK.

Printed by Fine Print (Services) Ltd, Oxford, UK.

Glossary

Android obesity: male-pattern obesity, characterized by increased accumulation of abdominal adipose tissue

Apo B$_{100}$: hepatic apolipoprotein B

Apo B$_{48}$: gut apolipoprotein B (its molecular weight is 48% that of apo B$_{100}$)

Apolipoproteins: structural proteins, often containing receptor binding sites

β-VLDL: chylomicron remnants and intermediate-density lipoprotein

CETP: cholesteryl ester transfer protein, which catalyses transfer of cholesterol from HDL to circulating triglyceride-rich lipoproteins, and from LDL back to VLDL

Cholesteryl ester: esterified cholesterol, which is more hydrophobic than free cholesterol

FH: familial hypercholesterolaemia

Foam cell: a cell, usually a macrophage, the cytoplasm of which has become loaded with cholesterol

Gynoid obesity: female-pattern obesity, characterized by increased depots in the buttocks and other peripheral sites

HDL: high-density lipoprotein

IDL: intermediate-density lipoprotein

LCAT: lecithin:cholesterol acyl transferase, which catalyses the esterification of free cholesterol

LDL: low-density lipoprotein

Lipaemia retinalis: pallor of the optic fundus and white appearance of the retinal veins and arteries due to extremely high levels of circulating chylomicrons

Lp(a): lipoprotein (a), an LDL-like particle that contains apolipoprotein (a) in addition to apo B

LpX: lipoprotein X, an abnormal lipoprotein present in plasma in obstructive jaundice

NEFA: non-esterified fatty acids

Small, dense LDL: cholesterol-depleted LDL that is not cleared through the LDL receptors, and is more atherogenic than normal LDL because it is readily oxidized

VLDL: very low-density lipoprotein

Introduction

In the space of a decade, the investigation and treatment of hyperlipidaemia has moved from being the eccentricity of a few academic specialists to occupy a position at the centre stage of everyday clinical practice. This is largely a result of the success of recent trials of lipid-lowering medication in decreasing the risk of coronary heart disease and stroke and, most importantly, extending life. This pace of progress has been reflected in the multitude of national and international guidelines for the prevention of cardiovascular disease, which have attempted to simplify the often complex issues surrounding the treatment of hyperlipidaemia. Clinical judgement cannot, however, be reduced to a set of tables. Instead, it relies on the ability of a physician to make a precise clinical diagnosis and to comprehend as fully as possible its causes and likely outcome in individual patients. We thus make no apology for providing a text that interprets clinical trial evidence in the context of pathogenesis and gives practical solutions to routine problems encountered in the clinical management of hyperlipidaemias.

CHAPTER 1
Lipids and lipoproteins

Cholesterol and triglycerides are the lipids most commonly measured in clinical practice. Although structurally diverse, all lipids are insoluble in water but soluble in non-polar solvents. For this reason, they tend to cling together in aqueous media, such as plasma, and thus to travel together. Their close physical association to avoid contact with water also leads to the most important structural role of lipids, the formation of cell membranes. The major components of cell membranes are cholesterol and phospholipids.

Triglycerides, however, constitute the ideal means of energy storage because of their exclusion from aqueous environments and their very high carbon content. The adipose cell is no more than a tiny rim of cytoplasm around a central droplet of energy-rich triglyceride (Figure 1.1), which, because of its insolubility, requires no water for storage. It is therefore light

(a)

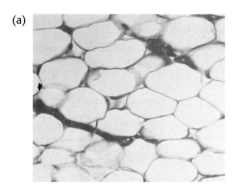

Figure 1.1 (a) Adipose cells. (b) A schematic showing the structural features.

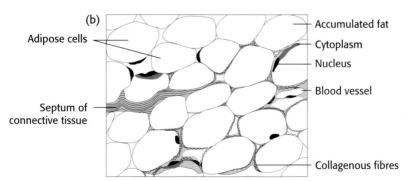

(b)

Adipose cells

Accumulated fat

Cytoplasm

Nucleus

Blood vessel

Septum of connective tissue

Collagenous fibres

in weight relative to its energy content compared with, for example, liver or muscle cells, which store relatively little energy in the form of carbohydrate (glycogen) per gram of tissue because of their high water content.

Cholesterol

Typical daily cholesterol intake is 200–500 mg (total dietary fat intake in countries such as the UK and the USA is probably 80–100 g/day). Cholesterol absorption from the gut is incomplete, with usually only around 30–60% of the quantity ingested actually entering the body. One of the paradoxes of human metabolism is that, although cholesterol is absorbed from the lumen of the gut, it is also secreted back into it as one of the components of bile. Furthermore, the body synthesizes at least as much as is obtained from the diet each day. Ideally, serum cholesterol should be below 5.0 mmol/litre (200 mg/dl).

The capacity to synthesize cholesterol is clearly important, as cholesterol is an essential component of cell membranes and is also the precursor for steroid hormones and vitamin D. Thus cholesterol synthesis within the body is essential during active growth or when dietary intake is limited, for example during famine or illness. However, the reason for cholesterol synthesis by well-nourished people without evident ill health is hard to explain. Cholesterol biosynthesis is increased with a high-energy diet and in obesity.

Almost all tissues can synthesize cholesterol, but much of its synthesis in the adult occurs in the liver, gut and central nervous system. Cholesterol biosynthesis, as one would expect, is extremely complex (Figure 1.2). However, an important physiological regulatory step occurs fairly early in the pathway, when 3-hydroxy-3-methylglutaryl CoA is converted to mevalonic acid. The enzyme responsible, HMG-CoA reductase, can be inhibited by a variety of physiological factors, the most important of which is probably the intracellular level of cholesterol. This is why tissues supplied with cholesterol in abundance from the liver and gut down-regulate their own cholesterol biosynthesis. The enzyme is also the site of action for the statin drugs (otherwise known as HMG-CoA reductase inhibitors).

Cholesterol can be free, with no fatty acid group attached to its OH group, or it can have a fatty acyl group bound by an ester link. For everyday

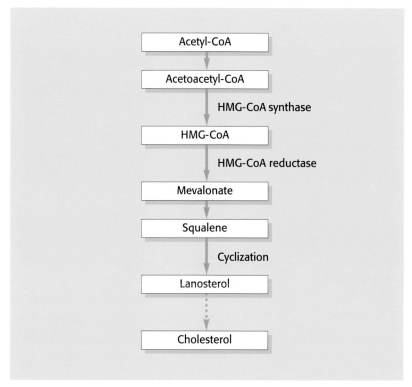

Figure 1.2 Cholesterol biosynthesis.

clinical purposes, the distinction between free and esterified cholesterol is not made and cholesterol values reported by the laboratory include both types. However, to understand the structure of a lipoprotein, it is necessary to know that the OH group of free cholesterol carries a slight electrical charge and so can interact with water to some extent, whereas esterified cholesterol has hardly any interaction with water.

Triglycerides

These constitute our major energy store. A reasonably lean adult man has about 15 kg of triglyceride, which yields about 38 kilojoules (9 Calories) for each gram respired. It thus represents an energy store of 570 000 kilojoules – roughly enough to survive starvation for 3 months. Most people have been taught that glycogen is an important energy store, and so it may be in the short term, but the body's store yields fewer than 4200 kilojoules and would thus be used up within the first day of starvation. Triglyceride is also the major energy source in human milk. Serum triglycerides are usually considered elevated if they exceed 2.3 mmol/litre (200 mg/dl) in the fasting state.

The adipose tissue in which triglyceride is stored performs other important roles. For example, because triglyceride is liquid at body temperature, the layers of fat around organs such as the kidneys (perinephric fascia) and in the omentum act as fluid cushions affording considerable protection. The subcutaneous adipose tissue not only accounts for much of the difference in physical appearance between men and women after puberty, but also provides a layer of thermal insulation.

Triglycerides undergo digestion in the gut to fatty acids and mono-glycerides. These are absorbed into the enterocytes and synthesized into chylomicrons for transport to the tissues. The liver can also synthesize triglycerides using fatty acids either from the circulation or synthesized from glucose. These triglycerides are assembled into lipoprotein particles, the very low-density lipoproteins (VLDL), and are released into the circulation.

When fatty acids are required to be released from adipose tissue stores, an intracellular enzyme, hormone-sensitive lipase, becomes active. Fatty acids are then released from the glycerol to which they are bound in the stored triglycerides. These fatty acids then move out of the adipose cell and, bound to albumin, are transported to other tissues. They are generally referred to as non-esterified fatty acids (NEFA). NEFA are released from adipose tissue during starvation (or the equivalent in affluent societies, namely a weight-reducing diet). One of the principal reasons for this is that hormone-sensitive lipase is inhibited by insulin and it thus becomes active when no food is entering the body and insulin levels are low. It is also activated by certain stress hormones, which also increase during starvation.

Some tissues, such as skeletal and cardiac muscle, can use circulating NEFA directly for respiration. However, many tissues lack the enzymes that break NEFA down to the 2-carbon acetyl-CoA necessary to enter the Krebs cycle and thus provide respiratory energy. The liver obligingly does this for them, producing ketone bodies (acetone, acetoacetate, 3-hydroxy-3-butyrate), which are water soluble and easily transported to the tissues where they can be simply converted to acetyl-CoA. This is why fasting makes the breath smell (the ketones are volatile) and why ketones in small amounts can be detected in the urine of many patients who are not eating. It is also the basis of the diabetic ketoacidosis that occurs when the pancreas is producing inadequate amounts of insulin to suppress the process: diabetic ketoacidosis is thus an inappropriate starvation response.

Phospholipids

These are the most highly charged of the lipids because of the presence of the phosphate group; they also often have other charged groups at the phosphate end of the molecule. The other end, however, is very similar to a triglyceride, comprising the long hydrocarbon sequences of fatty acyl groups. Thus one end of the molecule seeks water while the other orients itself towards non-polar substances, usually other lipids. This is essential for the role of phospholipids in membranes and lipoproteins.

Lipoprotein structure

Lipoproteins are macromolecular complexes of lipids (cholesterol, esterified cholesterol, triglycerides and phospholipids) and proteins (Figure 1.3). The protein components are apolipoproteins or enzymes. The apolipoproteins are structural proteins, which also often contain receptor binding sites, or proteins that modify the binding of other apolipoproteins to receptors. Thus the function of some apolipoproteins is to direct lipoproteins to particular tissues. Lipoproteins may also contain other lipid-soluble substances, such as vitamins, that are distributed around the body. Lipoproteins are mostly globular with a central core comprising a droplet of the most intensely hydrophobic lipids, the esterified cholesterol and triglycerides, surrounded by an outer shell in which free cholesterol is interspersed with phospholipids.

The principal sources of lipoproteins are the liver and gut, although it is being increasingly recognized that other tissues and organs can be a source of some of the apolipoprotein components.

Lipoprotein metabolism

Chylomicrons. The gut produces chylomicrons following absorption of the products of fat digestion (Figure 1.4). They are the largest of the lipoproteins and, in keeping with the composition of dietary fat, are richest in triglycerides. They are secreted initially into the lacteals of the villi and join the lymphatic circulation to enter the blood circulation via the thoracic

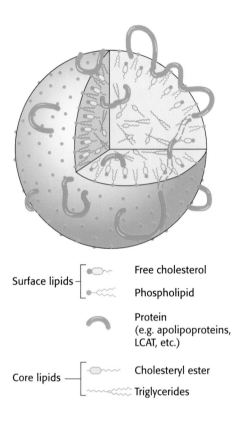

Free cholesterol

Phospholipid

Surface lipids

Protein
(e.g. apolipoproteins,
LCAT, etc.)

Cholesteryl ester

Core lipids

Triglycerides

Figure 1.3 The structure of a lipoprotein. The most hydrophobic components (the triglycerides and cholesteryl esters) form a central droplet, which is surrounded by the more polar components (free cholesterol, proteins and phospholipids). Proteins are arranged with their hydrophobic sequences inside the particle, while their hydrophilic regions are oriented towards the aqueous environment. The polar groups of cholesterol and phospholipids also point outwards, away from the hydrophobic core.

duct in the chest. Fat absorption is generally complete within a few hours of ingesting food, and the chylomicron concentration fluctuates during this time. Chylomicrons account for the postprandial rise in triglycerides, although this may be only modest in fit, healthy people. In others, however, the rise in triglycerides may be marked following the ingestion of food and may be prolonged if the clearance of chylomicrons from the circulation is delayed.

The triglyceride component of chylomicrons is removed by lipoprotein lipase. This enzyme is located on the vascular endothelium of tissues that have a high requirement for triglycerides as a source of energy or for storage, such as skeletal and cardiac muscle, adipose tissue and lactating breast. Lipoprotein lipase hydrolyses triglycerides to monoglycerides and fatty acids. The monoglycerides are broken down to glycerol and fatty acids by other tissue lipases. The resulting fatty acids and glycerol are then taken up by

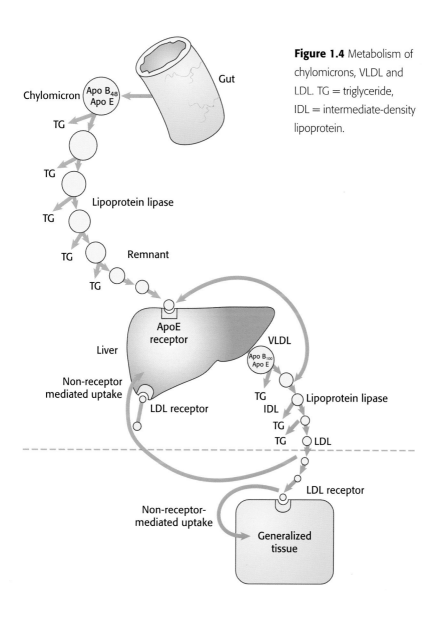

Figure 1.4 Metabolism of chylomicrons, VLDL and LDL. TG = triglyceride, IDL = intermediate-density lipoprotein.

cells and either respired or resynthesized into triglycerides for storage. The removal of triglycerides by lipoprotein lipase leaves chylomicron remnants in the circulation. These are removed by the liver via receptors that recognize apolipoprotein E (apo E).

Very low- and low-density lipoproteins. The hepatic triglyceride-rich lipoprotein is called very low-density lipoprotein (VLDL). Its triglycerides are removed by lipoprotein lipase during circulation. The smaller, less triglyceride-rich particle formed from VLDL is called low-density lipoprotein (LDL). Generally, the role of LDL is said to be to supply cholesterol to the tissues; this may be true under some circumstances, for example during growth and in tissues such as the adrenal gland or wounded tissues that continue to have a high requirement for cholesterol in adulthood. However, there is no obvious explanation for the high levels of LDL in the adult human. Serum LDL cholesterol in excess of 3.0 mmol/litre (120 mg/dl) and serum VLDL cholesterol concentrations in excess of 1.0 mmol/litre (40 mg/dl) are regarded as elevated.

LDL is certainly small enough to cross the capillary endothelium and enter the tissue fluid. When intracellular cholesterol pools become depleted, cells can synthesize a specialized receptor that migrates to the cell surface where it can combine with LDL in the tissue fluid. The receptor is then internalized in a pinocytotic vesicle and the cholesterol present in LDL is released into the cell. The receptor is termed the LDL receptor and mutations of it lead to familial hypercholesterolaemia (FH; see Chapter 3).

The heterogeneity in LDL particle composition, arising from differences in the amount of cholesterol per LDL particle, means that measuring LDL cholesterol is not equivalent to measuring LDL particle numbers. LDL may become depleted of cholesterol, and so patients with high levels of LDL may go undetected as neither total serum cholesterol nor LDL cholesterol measurements reflect the true LDL level. These points are important because increased concentrations of small, dense, cholesterol-depleted LDL particles are common in patients with vascular disease. Cholesterol-depleted LDL is not cleared through the LDL receptors, and is more atherogenic than its normal larger cousins. Small, dense LDL levels are often high in patients with hypertriglyceridaemia (be it primary or associated with, for example, diabetes) even when their serum cholesterol is low. The clue to the presence of small, dense LDL is low high-density lipoprotein (HDL) cholesterol.

High-density lipoprotein. About two-thirds to four-fifths of serum cholesterol is present in LDL. A small amount is present in VLDL, but most of the remainder is in HDL. HDL can receive excess cholesterol from the tissues and cholesterol can be transferred out of HDL to the liver and to other lipoproteins such as VLDL (Figure 1.5). Much of the cholesterol that HDL receives is unesterified and its capacity to continue to receive more is increased by the presence of an enzyme, lecithin:cholesterol acyl transferase (LCAT), which catalyses the esterification of free cholesterol. The cholesteryl ester so formed is even more intensely hydrophobic than free cholesterol; it can thus be packed tightly into the core of HDL while awaiting transfer out, allowing the HDL to pick up more free cholesterol.

Low levels of HDL are associated with an increased risk of coronary heart disease (CHD), and HDL is believed to have a protective role against

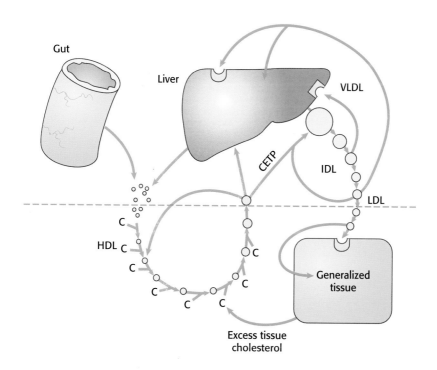

Figure 1.5 HDL is involved in reverse cholesterol transport. Excess cholesterol (C) from the tissues is released to HDL and is then either delivered to the liver or to VLDL in a process mediated by cholesteryl ester transfer protein (CETP). Some cholesteryl ester can be returned to the liver on LDL, but it can also find its way back to the tissues. IDL = intermediate-density lipoprotein.

atherosclerosis, perhaps because of its capacity to promote the transfer of cholesterol from tissues to the liver (reverse cholesterol transport). It has also recently been shown to protect LDL against atherogenic oxidative modification. Serum HDL cholesterol should exceed 0.9 mmol/litre (35 mg/dl).

HDL cholesterol levels are commonly low in hypertriglyceridaemia. This is partly because of a high rate of transfer of cholesterol from HDL, not to the liver, but to the large pool of circulating triglyceride-rich lipoproteins. This transfer is mediated by a transfer protein called cholesteryl ester transfer protein (CETP). A similar movement of cholesterol from LDL back to VLDL is also mediated by CETP, and the rate of this transfer is also increased in hypertriglyceridaemia (Figure 1.6).

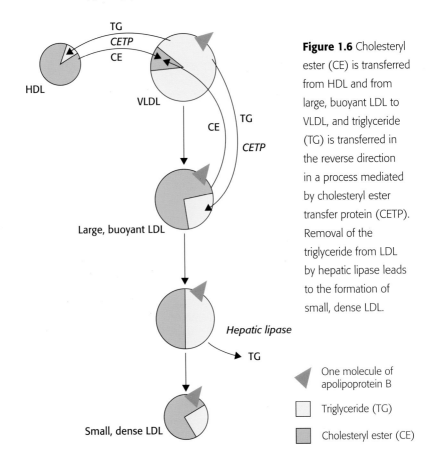

Figure 1.6 Cholesteryl ester (CE) is transferred from HDL and from large, buoyant LDL to VLDL, and triglyceride (TG) is transferred in the reverse direction in a process mediated by cholesteryl ester transfer protein (CETP). Removal of the triglyceride from LDL by hepatic lipase leads to the formation of small, dense LDL.

One molecule of apolipoprotein B

Triglyceride (TG)

Cholesteryl ester (CE)

Apolipoprotein B (apo B) is the apolipoprotein involved in chylomicron, VLDL and LDL metabolism. It is essential for the assembly and secretion of chylomicrons and VLDL, and also for the removal of LDL via the LDL receptor, because it is the part of LDL that is recognized by the LDL receptor. Interestingly, the apo B produced by the gut is shorter than that made in the liver. It contains the sequences necessary for chylomicron secretion, but lacks the part of the molecule recognized by the LDL receptor. This probably explains why chylomicron remnants are largely cleared by the liver, whereas LDL is free to provide cholesterol to the peripheral tissues. One consequence of this, however, is that LDL and the liver-derived apo B it contains are intimately involved in atherosclerosis. The hepatic apo B is called apo B_{100} and that from the gut apo B_{48} (because it only has 48% of the molecular weight of apo B_{100}).

CHAPTER 2
Epidemiology and pathophysiology

Lipids and coronary heart disease

Serum cholesterol concentration, reflecting LDL cholesterol concentration, is positively associated with the risk of CHD (Figure 2.1). This is true of just about every population studied, from the Chinese at the lowest end of the cholesterol scale to the British at the upper end. Serum HDL cholesterol concentration is inversely related to CHD risk.

Major differences exist between CHD rates around the world. In areas such as China, Indonesia, Japan and rural Africa, death from CHD is uncommon and generally occurs in old age, whereas in the USA, Canada, northern Europe, Australia and New Zealand, CHD is the most common cause of death from middle age onwards. Southern Europe has substantially

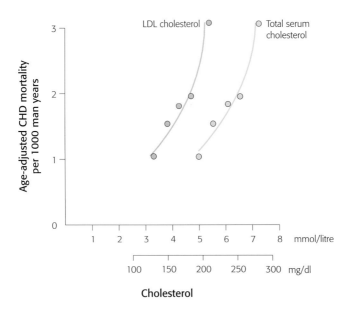

Figure 2.1 Relationship between CHD mortality and total serum cholesterol and LDL cholesterol. Data from Law MR *et al. BMJ* 1994;308:363–6.

lower CHD rates than northern Europe, although they are not as low as those generally found in Asia. The factor most closely related to CHD rates in Ancel Keys' Seven Countries Study was serum cholesterol; this observation has been confirmed, and an even closer relationship has been found using the serum cholesterol to HDL cholesterol ratio.

The diet in countries such as the UK has changed dramatically since the nineteenth century, when a substantial amount of dietary energy was, like those of countries with little CHD today, derived from carbohydrate (potatoes and cereal). Fat consumption, particularly in the forms of fatty meat and dairy products, has increased enormously this century. Obesity has also become more prevalent, not simply because of increased dietary energy intake, but also because of lower energy expenditure resulting from reduced physical activity and central heating.

The change in diet has paralleled the rise in incidence of CHD. Acute myocardial infarction was first described in 1911; although angina was well described in the eighteenth century, it is likely that much of this was not due to atheroma (i.e. it was probably the result of syphilis or valvular heart disease) or, if it was, it was relatively benign in that it was not associated with the acute thrombotic occlusion of coronary arteries. The increasing epidemic of CHD deaths between the 1920s and early 1980s reflected a genuine increase in coronary atheroma and thrombosis. In addition to nutritional changes, smoking cigarettes became popular during this time. Cigarettes were introduced into western Europe and thence the USA during the Crimean War. Although overall tobacco consumption in many countries has remained relatively static during this century, the proportion consumed as cigarettes has greatly increased.

CHD rates in countries with relatively high cholesterol levels correlate fairly well with cigarette consumption. However, the relationship disappears if countries with low cholesterol levels are also included: in Japan and China, cigarette smoking is common. It is also the case that, in countries with low mean serum cholesterol concentrations, people with other well-established risk factors for CHD in high-cholesterol countries (e.g. hypertension and diabetes) have a relatively lower risk. Therefore, in terms of cross-cultural epidemiology, cholesterol appears to be the permissive factor, without which the other risk factors have little impact.

Atherogenesis: events in the arterial wall

Anitschov, the great Russian experimental pathologist, wrote in 1913 that 'there can be no atheroma without cholesterol'. Just as the epidemiological evidence points firmly in that direction, so does our recent understanding of the pathological processes that lead to coronary atherogenesis, and subsequent thrombosis and occlusion. Disturbingly, in parts of the world with high CHD rates, the earliest lesions, which give rise to later atheroma, are prevalent among children. These early lesions are the fatty streaks that are commonly present in the aortas of children unfortunate enough to succumb to some unrelated sudden death, such as an accident. Fatty streaks consist of collections of cells loaded with cytoplasmic droplets of cholesterol beneath the intimal surface of an artery (Figure 2.2). These cells are called foam cells and are usually macrophages that have internalized LDL from the tissue fluid in such quantities as to load their cytoplasm with cholesterol droplets. The initiating event in fatty streak formation is the passage of increased quantities of LDL across the endothelium of an artery into its wall. This is likely to occur at sites of turbulence, where there may be relative anoxia, when LDL levels are high and when the endothelium is damaged by, for example, hypertension, oxidation or glycation. Monocytes from the blood circulation are attracted to these sites by the damaged endothelium and themselves cross the endothelium to enter the subintimal space, where they take up LDL and assume the morphology of macrophages. Healthy, unmodified LDL is taken up only slowly, if at all, by macrophages. It must undergo some modification before it can excite foam cell formation. The modification that has attracted most recent interest has been oxidation.

Oxidation. Oxygen is two electrons short of having the same electron shell as inert neon. It forms stable compounds by sharing electrons from the outer shells of the atoms with which it reacts – for example, one from each of two hydrogen atoms to form water. Reactions of oxygen, including those catalysed by enzymes, involve the production of an intermediate in which oxygen has acquired one additional electron in its outer shell, but has yet to receive the second to complete the reaction. At this stage, it is known as an oxygen free radical and is highly reactive, with its outer electron shell resembling that of fluorine. Oxygen free radicals are particularly reactive at the site of double carbon bonds in organic

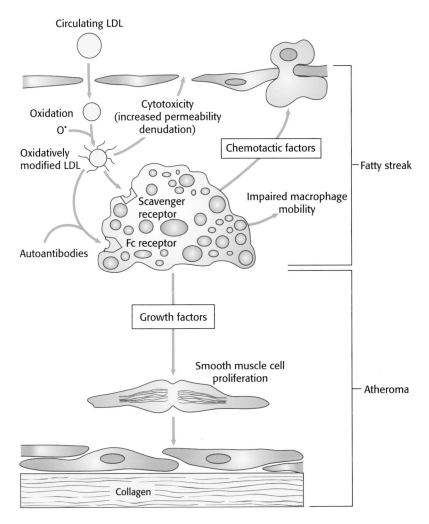

Figure 2.2 Atherogenesis: the fatty streak is characterized by lipid-laden macrophages (foam cells derived from blood monocytes attracted to the arterial subintima, where they engulf lipoproteins, such as oxidatively modified LDL). Conversion of the fatty streak to atheroma depends on the proliferation and differentiation of smooth-muscle cells into fibroblasts, the elaboration of collagen and repetition of the whole process. As the lesion progresses, necrosis of foam cells leaves behind extracellular lipid deposits; an overlying fibrous cap develops (see Figure 2.4). The actively growing point of the lesion where new foam cells are forming is in the shoulder at the junction between the atheromatous lesion and the normal arterial wall.

compounds. LDL has an abundance of these in the fatty acids of the phospholipids present in its outer envelope. Oxygen free-radical attack on these phospholipids leads to the formation of lipid peroxidation products. These react with, and damage, the apo B of LDL, altering its receptor-binding characteristics. This oxidatively modified LDL is rapidly taken up by macrophages through a class of receptors called scavenger receptors to form foam cells.

Oxygen free radicals:
- are present in cigarette smoke
- are formed during glycation reactions
- are generated deliberately by macrophages, for example to kill bacteria
- may leak from a variety of oxidative pathways.

Antioxidant mechanisms. LDL has its own fat-soluble antioxidants, which are dissolved in its central lipid droplet. They include:
- ubiquinone
- vitamin E (α- and β-tocopherol)
- β-carotene.

These are chain-breaking antioxidants; they themselves react more readily with oxygen free radicals than phospholipids. Despite the widescale consumption of vitamin E and β-carotene in the belief that they will protect against atheroma, clinical evidence of such an effect is not entirely convincing. This is perhaps because when fat-soluble antioxidants are themselves oxidized, they offer no further protection against oxidation and may even behave as pro-oxidants. Water-soluble antioxidant vitamins, such as vitamin C, to which fat-soluble antioxidants can pass the oxygen free radicals they have reacted with, may thus be critical.

HDL also appears to protect LDL against oxidative modification. It does so not by interfering with the formation of lipid peroxides on LDL, but by metabolizing them before they undergo spontaneous breakdown to form apo B-damaging substances. A means of enhancing this activity is as yet unknown – the best policy for decreasing the production of oxidatively modified LDL is to reduce the quantity of LDL present in the circulation, or at least that of the subfractions of LDL which are most susceptible to oxidation.

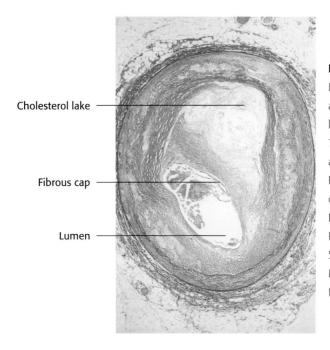

Cholesterol lake

Fibrous cap

Lumen

Figure 2.3
Mature atheromatous lesion occluding 70% of the arterial lumen. Reproduced courtesy of the Department of Pathological Sciences, Manchester Royal Infirmary, UK.

Effects of oxidatively modified LDL. These are not confined to foam cell formation. Oxidatively modified LDL can also directly damage endothelial cells, stimulate the formation of autoantibodies, and excite macrophages and endothelial cells to secrete chemotactic factors that attract circulating monocytes. Foam cells themselves can produce growth factors that recruit smooth-muscle cells located further out in the aortic wall into the fatty streak region. These smooth-muscle cells differentiate into fibroblasts and lay down collagen. This response, which is clearly part of an inappropriately activated tissue repair process, leads to the development of the atheromatous plaque, the mature atheromatous lesion (Figure 2.3).

Plaque formation. The collagen elaborated by fibroblasts comes to overlie the macrophage foam cells, which undergo either necrosis or apoptosis. This results in the formation of a pool of extracellular cholesterol trapped beneath a fibrous cap. The shoulder of the atheromatous lesion (where the fibrous cap joins the normal arterial wall) continues to be active and it is here that active foam cell formation continues as the lesion advances across the inner surface of the artery (Figure 2.4). The fibrous cap is also at its most

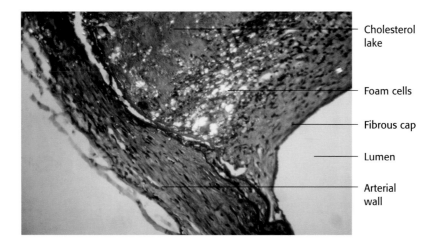

Cholesterol lake

Foam cells

Fibrous cap

Lumen

Arterial wall

Figure 2.4 The active shoulder region of a mature, cholesterol-rich plaque. At this site, the foam cells are clearly active (the orange-red material is lipid stained with Oil Red O, and pale intracellular cholesterol crystals are also present within the macrophages) and the fibrous cap is most vulnerable to rupture. Reproduced courtesy of the Department of Pathological Sciences, Manchester Royal Infirmary, UK.

mechanically weak in this region; the secretion of collagenase from the macrophage foam cells may exacerbate this weakness. The part of the cap that ruptures is almost invariably in the shoulder of the plaque. Cholesterol-rich plaques are particularly liable to rupture their overlying fibrous cap. This becomes less likely as the quantity of fibrous tissue binding down the cap increases. Asymptomatic lesions, which occlude only 40–50% of the coronary artery lumen at a stage when they are particularly rich in cholesterol, may be more liable to rupture their caps than larger more fibrous lesions that obstruct the artery sufficiently to cause stable angina.

Rupture of a fibrous cap may lead to discharge of the cholesterol lake from beneath it. Should healing of the broken surface then occur uneventfully, a largely fibrous atheromatous lesion will result. However, if the victim of plaque rupture is unfortunate, thrombosis will occur at the raw site of the ruptured cap (Figure 2.5). Extension of this thrombosis will cause acute occlusion of the coronary artery lumen, resulting in myocardial infarction or unstable angina.

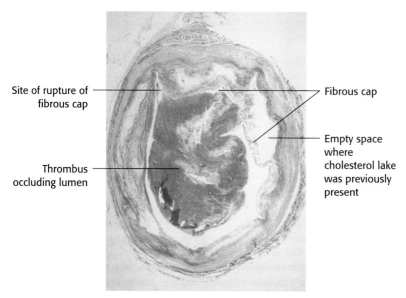

Site of rupture of fibrous cap

Fibrous cap

Empty space where cholesterol lake was previously present

Thrombus occluding lumen

Figure 2.5 A ruptured plaque discharging the cholesterol lake beneath the fibrous cap. Thrombus has formed at the raw endothelial surface of the rupture site and the lumen is completely occluded. Reproduced courtesy of the Department of Pathological Sciences, Manchester Royal Infirmary, UK.

Factors that may ultimately determine the fate of a person harbouring coronary atheroma include:

- those promoting plaque rupture, such as a high circulating concentration of LDL cholesterol (contributing to formation of plaques enriched in cholesterol relative to collagen and heightening foam cell activity in the vulnerable parts of the plaque and/or sudden rises in blood pressure)
- those that make thrombosis more likely, such as cigarette smoking and diabetes, which increase circulating plasma fibrinogen levels
- the extent of myocardial damage when occlusion occurs or the propensity of the ischaemic myocardium to dysrhythmia.

The scale of the problem

The UK population probably has the highest serum cholesterol levels in the world. CHD rates in the west of Scotland and Northern Ireland have recently been exceeded by those of the Czech Republic, so it is possible that other countries are in contention. Nevertheless, it is probably the worst single cause of ill health and premature death in the UK. Two-thirds of the UK population have serum cholesterol levels exceeding the optimal upper limit for a population, 5.2 mmol/litre. The situation is better in the USA (Table 2.1), where both serum cholesterol and CHD rates are lower. They are not, however, sufficiently low that there can be any grounds for complacency.

A note on classification of hyperlipoproteinaemias

The World Health Organization (WHO) or, as it was more popularly known, Frederickson classification of the hyperlipoproteinaemias (Table 2.2)

TABLE 2.1

Serum cholesterol levels in the UK and USA

	Serum cholesterol mmol/litre (mg/dl)			
	UK*		USA**	
Age (years)	Median	90th percentile	Median	90th percentile
Men				
0–24	–	–	4.0 (154)	5.0 (193)
25–34	5.4 (208)	6.8 (262)	4.8 (185)	6.1 (235)
35–44	6.0 (231)	7.5 (289)	5.3 (205)	6.4 (260)
45–75	6.2 (239)	7.8 (300)	5.6 (215)	7.0 (270)
75+	5.9 (227)	7.4 (285)	5.3 (204)	6.6 (255)
Women				
0–24	–	–	4.1 (158)	4.9 (189)
25–34	5.2 (200)	6.4 (247)	4.7 (180)	6.0 (230)
35–44	5.5 (212)	6.7 (257)	4.9 (190)	6.2 (240)
45–55	6.1 (235)	7.5 (289)	5.5 (212)	7.3 (280)
55+	6.8 (262)	8.5 (327)	6.0 (230)	7.5 (290)

*From Dong et al. Health Survey for England 1994. London: HMSO, 1996:369–419
**From Rifkin BM, Segal P. Lipid Research Clinics Program reference values of hyperlipidaemia and hypolipidaemia. JAMA 1983;250:1869–72 and National Health and Nutrition Examination Survey (NHANES) III Data

TABLE 2.2

WHO classification of hyperlipoproteinaemias

Type	Lipoprotein(s) elevated	Lipid(s) elevated
I	Chylomicrons	Triglycerides and cholesterol
IIa	LDL	Cholesterol
IIb	VLDL and LDL	Cholesterol and triglycerides
III	β-VLDL	Triglycerides and cholesterol
IV	VLDL	Triglycerides
V	Chylomicrons and VLDL	Triglycerides and cholesterol

is still commonly used. It is not a diagnostic classification and does not give any indication of prognosis. Type IIa hyperlipoproteinaemia includes, for example, both FH, which untreated often leads to morbidity and premature death, and mild polygenic hypercholesterolaemia, which in a patient with a high HDL cholesterol and no other risk factors may be entirely harmless. WHO typing is simply a biochemical phenotypic classification based on which lipoprotein level is raised. It was devised before the importance of HDL cholesterol as a prognostic indicator was appreciated. It refers therefore to only three of the classes of lipoprotein so far discussed, chylomicrons, VLDL and LDL, and to one class of lipoprotein, β-VLDL, which occurs only pathologically (see page 57).

CHAPTER 3
Familial (monogenic) hypercholesterolaemia

Heterozygous familial hypercholesterolaemia

Genetic basis. FH is the most common genetic disorder in Europe and the USA, affecting about 1 in 500 people in its heterozygous form. The existence of a dominantly inherited form of hypercholesterolaemia causing tendon xanthomata has been recognized for 70 years. The nature of the genetic mutation causing the condition was not revealed, however, until 1974 when Goldstein and Brown in Dallas discovered the LDL receptor and found its expression to be diminished in fibroblasts from patients with FH. It is now known that the gene for the LDL receptor is located on chromosome 19.

The LDL receptor allows LDL to be taken up by cells from the tissue fluid. Newly synthesized receptors migrate to the cell surface where they can bind LDL. They move through the cell membrane to the region of the cell surface containing the coated pits, where invagination of the cell membrane is active. The invaginated membrane enters the cell cytoplasm as a vesicle containing a whole variety of receptors and their bound ligands. In the case of the LDL receptors, these are released back into the cytoplasm leaving any LDL they are carrying behind in the vesicle. They then travel back to the cell membrane so that the whole cycle may be repeated. This is believed to occur about every 10 minutes. The vesicles containing LDL fuse to form larger vesicles, called endosomes, into which enzymes are secreted that break down the apo B and esterified cholesterol to amino acids and free cholesterol, respectively; these can then diffuse out into the cytoplasm.

In FH, a mutation of the receptor prevents it from participating efficiently in LDL uptake, because it cannot be transported to the cell surface, cannot bind properly to LDL once it gets there, cannot be internalized, or is not released from the endosome. In FH heterozygotes, one of the LDL-receptor genes has a mutation; in homozygous FH, both do. Well before the discovery of the LDL-receptor defect, it was shown that the time LDL spent in the circulation before its removal was increased from the normal 2.5 days to about 4.5 days in heterozygotes and even longer in homozygotes (Figure 3.1). Impaired LDL uptake is the basis of this observation.

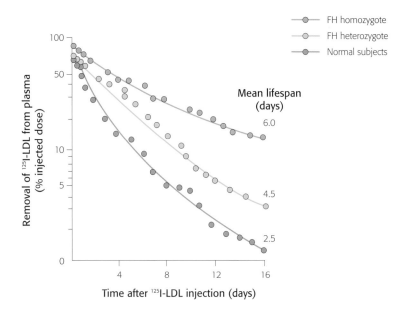

Figure 3.1 Radiolabelled LDL disappears from the circulation more slowly in patients with familial hypercholesterolaemia than in normal controls. Data from Bilheimer *et al. J Clin Invest* 1979;64:524–33.

A wide variety of mutations of the LDL receptor have been found to cause the clinical syndrome of FH in societies such as the UK and USA – more than 200 have been reported. In societies that have arisen relatively recently from a small number of early settlers or migrants, the frequency of FH may be more than 1 in 500, and it will be caused by a smaller number of different mutations. For example, 1 in 80 South Africans of Dutch or French descent have FH and the majority have one of only three different LDL-receptor mutations. Two of the mutations can be traced back to two of the early Dutch settlers and the other to a Huguenot migrant. A similar situation appears to exist among descendants of French Canadian settlers, and the high prevalence of FH in the Lebanon has sometimes been ascribed to an LDL-receptor mutation introduced by a Crusader. In families with members affected by FH, marriage to close relatives for cultural or religious reasons is also likely to increase greatly the likelihood of producing a family member with homozygous FH.

Diagnosis. FH can generally be diagnosed with ease if features of the clinical syndrome are carefully sought in people with hypercholesterolaemia. Whether the FH genotype can be present in people without the clinical syndrome is debatable, as is the role of genetic testing. It seems highly likely, however, that people with the FH genotype and no clinical features of FH are rare and it is by no means certain that they are at risk of premature CHD. Furthermore, because of the variety of mutations encountered in unrelated patients with FH, no simple, widely applicable means of genetic testing is feasible, except perhaps in a country such as South Africa where a much smaller number of different mutations exist.

It is important to emphasize that the introduction of lipid-lowering therapy is not the only reason for identifying heterozygotes for FH. The disorder is still not widely recognized. Therefore, when FH patients present with manifestations of CHD, they are often inappropriately managed if seen by physicians unfamiliar with the condition. There is a general disbelief that apparently fit, young people can have severe CHD. This usually leads to delay in investigations, particularly coronary angiography. Certainly exercise electrocardiography should be carried out promptly should symptoms that are, in the least, suggestive of CHD occur and FH patients should be encouraged to report such symptoms. Coronary angiograms often reveal surprisingly extensive disease despite relatively minimal symptoms and should not be withheld. The pressure gradient across the aortic valve should be measured using echocardiography when a systolic murmur is present.

Cholesterol measurements. Serum cholesterol in heterozygous FH is raised from birth – normal mean serum cholesterol concentration in umbilical cord blood is only 1.7–2.0 mmol/litre (65–80 mg/dl). However, screening using total serum cholesterol is not recommended at this stage because, in many babies without FH, high HDL cholesterol (the dominant lipoprotein in fetal blood) is a much more common cause of high cord-blood cholesterol levels than FH. Serum cholesterol rises in the first year of life to a mean of 4.1 mmol/litre (160 mg/dl; 95th percentile, 5.2 mmol/litre or 200 mg/dl) and persists until the early teens with mean levels being similar in boys and girls before puberty. The normal range for serum cholesterol varies little with age during childhood; this allows a diagnostic threshold for childhood FH to be defined and explains why a total serum cholesterol above 6.7 mmol/litre (260 mg/dl) identifies 95% of heterozygotes and only

2.5% of unaffected children. It is, of course, important to confine cholesterol measurements to the children of affected parents, so that the chances of the condition occurring are 1 in 2. If children in general were screened, the chance of finding a heterozygote would be 1 in 500, so even a 2.5% false-positive rate would falsely identify ten unaffected children for every one affected. In almost all affected children, the serum cholesterol exceeds 7.0 mmol/litre (270 mg/dl). In families with FH, measuring cholesterol in childhood can lead to uncertainty if serum cholesterol is 5.5–7.0 mmol/litre (210–270 mg/dl), particularly if the family is already on a cholesterol-lowering diet. The diagnosis cannot then be made or excluded with complete confidence, and repeated measurements over time are required.

With advancing age, the serum cholesterol in FH, as in the general population, increases. In heterozygous FH, it is generally double what it would have been in the absence of the LDL-receptor mutation. For example, in a young adult woman whose serum cholesterol might have been only 4.0 mmol/litre (150 mg/dl) had she not inherited the disorder, a level of 8.0 mmol/litre (300 mg/dl) may indicate FH. By adulthood, the serum cholesterol in heterozygous FH is, however, typically in the range 9.0–14.0 mmol/litre (350–550 mg/dl).

Tendon xanthomata, corneal arcus and xanthelasmata. Tendon xanthomata are the diagnostic hallmarks of FH. The only other causes of these, cerebrotendinous xanthomata and phytosterolaemia, are so rare that, for practical purposes, in the presence of tendon xanthomata, the diagnosis of FH is never really in doubt. Xanthomata are localized infiltrates of lipid-containing foam cells that histologically resemble atheroma.

Corneal arcus (Figure 3.2) and xanthelasmata (Figure 3.3) are not specific for FH, though they often occur much earlier in life in people with FH than in those with the more common polygenic type of hypercholesterolaemia (see Chapter 4). Corneal arcus, for example, in the late teens or twenties may well indicate FH. On the other hand, xanthelasmata not infrequently occur in women during their first pregnancy when, at other times, their serum cholesterol is not particularly high. A great many FH heterozygotes with obvious tendon xanthomata do not have corneal arcus until much later, however, and will never develop xanthelasmata. Tendon xanthomata should, therefore, be sought in all patients with hypercholesterolaemia, regardless of the presence of corneal arcus or xanthelasmata. 31

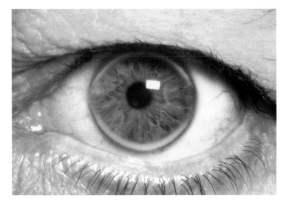

Figure 3.2 Corneal arcus.

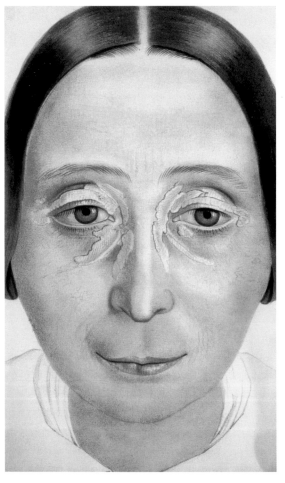

Figure 3.3 Eliza Parachute, the first patient described with xanthelasmata (Addison & Gull Guy's Hospital Reports 1851;series II, 7:265–70).

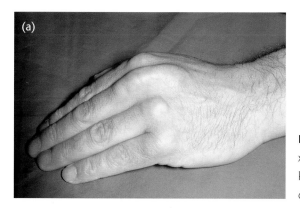

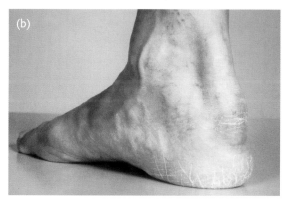

Figure 3.4 Tendon xanthomata on (a) the knuckle, reproduced courtesy of Dr JH Barth, Leeds General Infirmary, UK, and (b) the Achilles tendon.

The most common sites for tendon xanthomata are in the tendons overlying the knuckles and in the Achilles tendons (Figure 3.4). Less commonly, they may be found in the extensor hallucis longus and triceps tendons, and occasionally others. It is quite common to find xanthomata on the tibial tuberosity at the site of insertion of the patellar tendon (Figure 3.5). These are called subperiosteal xanthomata and are firmly attached to the bone.

It must be emphasized that the skin overlying tendon xanthomata and subperiosteal xanthomata has a normal colour and does not appear yellow. The cholesterol accumulation is deep within the tendons and much of the swelling is fibrous. The xanthomata feel hard. Those in the Achilles tendons show a tendency to become inflamed and many patients with FH will, if asked, give a history of earlier episodes of Achilles tenosynovitis. Xanthomata in the tendons on the dorsum of the hands are generally nodular or fusiform

33

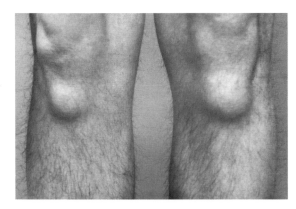

Figure 3.5
Subperiosteal
xanthomata over
tibial tuberosities.

and, because they often overlie the knuckles (particularly when the fist is clenched) and are as hard as bone, physicians may miss them. The hand should be examined with the fingers extended – the xanthomata move back and can be moved from side to side. Achilles tendon xanthomata may be obvious, if sought, because of thickening, swelling, irregularity or nodularity of the tendon on visual inspection. They may, however, be more subtle with the nodularity on the tendon only becoming obvious on palpation.

Family history. The other striking feature of FH is often the adverse family history of CHD, though sadly, of course, in societies like those of northern Europe and North America, a family history of early-onset CHD is common in the general population. Nonetheless, because FH is treatable, its diagnosis should always be sought when such a history is encountered. It is hypercholesterolaemia that is inherited in FH, not necessarily the propensity to premature CHD. In some families, FH seems particularly devastating, causing CHD in men in their twenties and women before the menopause. In others, men are unaffected until late middle age and occasionally older, and women may survive to extreme old age with minimal CHD symptoms.

The general level of CHD risk can be appreciated from Table 3.1. The median age for the development of CHD in men is around 50 years. Typically, affected women in the same family develop CHD about 9 years later than their male relatives with FH. Furthermore, the penetrance of FH judged in terms of CHD risk tends to breed true in families. Thus it is striking how often one encounters a family in whom all the affected male members developed CHD at a similar age and their affected female relatives some

TABLE 3.1

CHD incidence and mortality associated with untreated heterozygous FH*

Age (years)	CHD incidence (%)		CHD mortality (%)	
	Men	Women	Men	Women
< 30	5	0	0	0
30–39	22	2	7	0
40–49	48	7	25	1
50–59	80	51	52	15
60–69	100	75	78	23

*Compilation of studies in the UK (Slack. *Lancet* 1969;2:1380–2), the USA (Stone *et al. Circulation* 1974;49:476–88) and France (Beaumont *et al. Atherosclerosis* 1976;24:441–50)

9 years later. This can be helpful clinically – for example, in making decisions as to the age at which to introduce lipid-lowering medication. If the family history is particularly adverse, this might be as early as adolescence in male heterozygotes. In other families in which the hypercholesterolaemia is pursuing a more benign course, medication may be started later; for example, in many women from such families, the introduction of cholesterol-lowering medication can safely be left until they are in their thirties or later.

Tenosynositis. In addition to Achilles tendonitis, a more generalized tenosynositis may occur in FH. This is most commonly seen when cholesterol is lowered abruptly by, for example, partial ileal bypass, but it can also occur when cholesterol is lowered with other therapies, such as statins, when it may be wrongly attributed to the drug itself. It is due to the mobilization of cholesterol widely deposited in the tendons and periarticular tissues, and is akin to the exacerbations of gout that may accompany the mobilization of uric acid when allopurinol is introduced for the first time.

Homozygous familial hypercholesterolaemia

This is rare when it occurs by chance. The odds of two unrelated heterozygotes marrying is 1 in 250 000 (unless, of course, they meet at a lipid clinic) and the chances of them having a child who is homozygous is

1 in 4, making the theoretical incidence of homozygous FH 1 in a million.
The chances of a marriage between heterozygotes is greatly increased
when there is, for example, a tradition of first-cousin marriage. In such
circumstances, both of the LDL-receptor mutations in homozygotes are
likely to be the same, and the affected person is a true homozygote.
Homozygotes arising from random union are likely to have a different
LDL-receptor mutation on each chromosome and are, in reality, compound
heterozygotes (though they are classified as homozygotes).

Signs. Homozygous FH is always a serious problem. Serum cholesterol levels
are almost invariably greater than 15 mmol/litre (600 mg/dl) and can be as
high as 30 mmol/litre (1200 mg/dl). Xanthomata develop in childhood. In
addition to florid tendon xanthomata of the type already described, orange-
yellow cutaneous planar xanthomata develop, particularly in the popliteal
and antecubital fossae, buttocks and in the webs between the fingers
(Figure 3.6). They may develop on the palms of the hands and the fronts of
the knees during crawling. Polyarthralgia is common and supravalvar aortic
stenosis can cause sudden death. Most homozygotes develop angina of effort
in childhood due to the aortic stenosis and coronary atheroma. Myocardial
infarction has been recorded as early as at 2 years and life expectancy does
not usually extend beyond the early twenties. The very worst prognosis
seems to occur when both LDL-receptor mutations are of the type that
completely prevents LDL receptors appearing on the cell surface.

Management

Heterozygous FH. The statin drugs represent a major advance in the
management of FH. Most people with heterozygous FH can now achieve
serum cholesterol levels below 7.0 mmol/litre (270 mg/dl) and some even
below 5.0 mmol/litre (200 mg/dl). The most potent of the statins may be
required at maximum dose in patients with the higher cholesterol levels.
Occasionally the therapeutic response is still inadequate, in which case a
bile-acid sequestrating agent is the most logical addition. Nicotinic acid in
doses up to 7 g daily is also effective, but must be carefully monitored and
is rarely acceptable to patients because of the severe flushing it invariably
produces. Partial ileal bypass is often successful in decreasing serum
cholesterol, but has been used less often since the advent of statins.

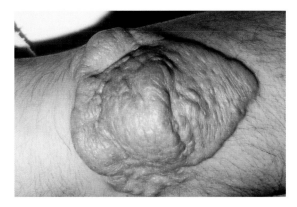

Figure 3.6

Subcutaneous planar xanthoma in the antecubital fossa. Reproduced courtesy of Dr JP Miller, University Hospital of South Manchester, UK.

Homozygous FH. The cholesterol-lowering effect achieved with medication in homozygous FH is generally disappointing, with the exception of that achieved with atorvastatin, which can decrease serum cholesterol by up to 30%. Even then, substantial hypercholesterolaemia remains. Plasmapheresis or LDL apheresis is the best approach to correcting this. Generally the procedure must be carried out every 2 weeks. Liver transplantation has also met with some success. This introduces normal donor hepatic LDL receptors. The LDL-receptor gene can be expressed in transfected LDL-receptor knockout mice, lowering serum cholesterol albeit only briefly before it is cleared from the cell nuclei along with viral DNA. Homozygous FH will be one of the first genetic disorders to be treated by this technique as soon as a vector that allows foreign DNA to persist in mammalian cells becomes available.

Genetic counselling

There is no need to suggest that a patient with heterozygous FH should limit their family as long as their partner is not also a heterozygote. It is advisable to check the partner's serum cholesterol to establish this. Although one child in two of a heterozygote for FH with a non-FH partner will themselves be FH heterozygotes, the prospect for improved treatment is great and the condition not generally so severe as to believe that such individuals will not benefit from their life. However, depending on the family history, it may be sensible that FH patients do not wait until the bloom of youth is too far behind them before starting their families, because of the devastating effect the death of a parent can have on young children.

Familial defective apo B

The FH phenotype is usually caused by an LDL-receptor mutation. Rarely, however, the same FH syndrome is caused because apo B has a mutation that interferes with binding, thus producing a similar defect in LDL catabolism. This is called familial defective apo B (FDB). It is most commonly due to an amino-acid substitution at position 3500. This mutation has a frequency of about 1 in 600 in the general population, though it does not generally produce a particularly severe hyperlipidaemia. It has, however, been estimated that perhaps as many as 4% of people with clinical FH have FDB. Their hypercholesterolaemia appears to respond more easily to treatment than is generally the case in FH.

Other mutations leading to FH

Currently, about half of the patients in the UK and USA with a clinical diagnosis of heterozygous FH will have identifiable mutations of the LDL receptor; a much smaller proportion will have FDB. It is possible that genetic techniques are failing to detect LDL-receptor mutations in some FH patients. It is also possible that another gene or genes involved in LDL catabolism will be found that, when they undergo mutation, explain the presence of FH in some patients. Although this adds considerable interest to the subject, we already have sufficient knowledge of the natural history of the clinical syndrome of FH to treat it with vigour.

CHD susceptibility

CHD is far and away the most common manifestation of atheroma in heterozygous FH. Atheromatous deposits may also occur in the root of the aorta and can extend into the aortic valve cusps; these occur particularly in homozygous FH, but also in as many as 30% of heterozygotes. This form of supravalvar aortic stenosis and aortic sclerosis may be the cause of an aortic systolic murmur. Some patients also develop carotid and intracerebral atheroma, though not as frequently as CHD. Femoropopliteal atheroma is also less common than CHD and is really only encountered in cigarette smokers with FH.

There has been much speculation as to why some families with FH are more susceptible to CHD than others. The nature of the mutation might itself be important, because some mutations will more severely compromise

LDL uptake than others. The particular combination of mutations certainly influences the severity of homozygous FH, but this is less clear in hetero-zygous FH. Indeed, neither the pre-treatment LDL cholesterol level nor the extent and size of tendon xanthomata is clearly related to prognosis in FH. Serum HDL cholesterol is, however, related to the likelihood of CHD in FH. Serum HDL cholesterol is generally lower than expected in FH; prognosis is often bad in families where this is most obvious. Usually in FH, only the serum cholesterol is raised as a consequence of the increase in LDL. Triglycerides are elevated in a minority of patients, though seldom to more than 4.0 mmol/litre (350 mg/dl). This too has been associated with a worse prognosis. These people are often obese and obesity can increase serum cholesterol, sometimes even to 20 mmol/litre (800 mg/dl) or more.

Obesity is generally uncommon in FH, in contrast to all other hyper-lipidaemias in which obesity is over-represented. Hypertension and diabetes mellitus are noticeably uncommon in FH; again, this is unlike other hyper-lipoproteinaemias. Cigarette smoking may be more common in some families with a worse prognosis and socio-economic deprivation almost certainly worsens the outlook.

CHAPTER 4
Polygenic and familial combined hyperlipidaemias

In the UK and USA, FH, though extremely important to detect and treat, is not the most common cause of hypercholesterolaemia. The great majority of people with raised serum cholesterol levels will have polygenic hyper-cholesterolaemia; like height, this is the consequence of several genes and their interaction with acquired, largely nutritional, factors.

Polygenic hypercholesterolaemia

When FH can be diagnosed, either because hypercholesterolaemia is present in childhood or an adult has the clinical features of the syndrome, a reasonably accurate estimate of clinical risk can be made and appropriate therapy given. In the UK, however, FH probably accounts for no more than 3% of men dying of CHD before the age of 60. Overlap exists between the range of LDL cholesterol levels encountered in FH and those due to polygenic hypercholesterolaemia, though in the latter they are generally lower.

Estimates of the contribution of different levels of cholesterol on the overall cumulative male mortality from CHD are given in Table 4.1. The majority of these premature deaths come from the middle part of the cholesterol distribution, and therefore it has been argued that, if a significant reduction in the incidence of CHD is to be achieved in countries such as the UK, efforts to lower cholesterol cannot simply be confined to those individuals whose serum cholesterol measurements lie at the upper end of the distribution. Nevertheless, because the number of people in the middle range is so huge (the vast majority of whom are not at increased risk of premature CHD), a non-clinical cholesterol-lowering strategy is appropriate for them. This is the 'low-risk' or 'population' strategy, which aims to lower serum cholesterol via public health measures aimed at encouraging the adoption of a lower fat diet and the avoidance of obesity.

Risk factors. Some patients from the middle range of cholesterol are, however, at much greater individual risk from their cholesterol level than the majority, because they have other risk factors for CHD that increase their susceptibility. Probably the most potent of these is that the individual already

TABLE 4.1

Relationship between serum cholesterol and risk of premature CHD death in UK men

Serum cholesterol level	Risk of death before 60 years (per 1000)	Population with the cholesterol level (%)	Population dying before the age of 60 years with the cholesterol level (%)
< 5 mmol/litre (< 190 mg/dl)	25	10	0.25
5–6 mmol/litre (190–230 mg/dl)	30	35	1.05
6–7 mmol/litre (230–270 mg/dl)	43	40	1.72
7–8 mmol/litre (270–310 mg/dl)	55	10	0.55
8–9 mmol/litre (310–345 mg/dl)	74	4	0.30
> 9 mmol/litre (> 345 mg/dl)	130	1	0.13
Heterozygous FH	500	0.2	0.1
Total			**4.1**

has CHD. In middle-aged myocardial-infarction survivors, serum cholesterol is an important indicator of prognosis (Figure 4.1), ranking after left ventricular insufficiency, but ahead of most of the other risk factors for CHD. Inappropriate lipoprotein levels are also the most important risk factors for occlusion of coronary artery bypass grafts after the initial postoperative period. In people who have not yet developed CHD, the effect of risk factors such as cigarette smoking, hypertension and diabetes is also to increase the risk from any given level of cholesterol (Figure 4.2). A family history of CHD at an early age in a first-degree relative also increases the likelihood of CHD, and part of this effect is independent of other risk factors. The combination of these factors with a relatively modestly increased serum cholesterol level can increase individual risk substantially, and to a level at which clinical intervention is justified. Identification and

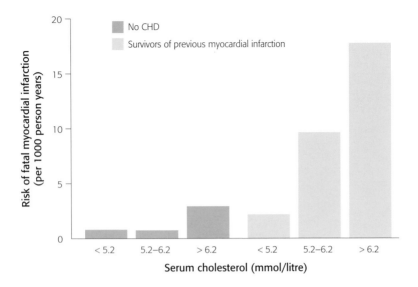

Figure 4.1 The risk of subsequent fatal myocardial infarction in survivors of myocardial infarction and in those without clinically evident CHD, according to serum cholesterol. Data from Pekkanen *et al. N Engl J Med* 1990;322:1700–7.

treatment of such people constitutes the 'high-risk' or clinical approach to CHD prevention.

Management. The intensity with which the clinician should intervene is probably best estimated with regard to an absolute risk (see Figure 10.1, pages 98–99). The use of absolute CHD risk as the sole arbiter of whether or not to introduce lipid-lowering medication does, however, have the effect of directing treatment towards patients in an older age range. This may be appropriate, but it can mean that statin treatment is used at risk levels which are no more than average in the elderly while people in their thirties, whose CHD risk is 100 times that of the average person of that age, go untreated. All patients with hypercholesterolaemia should receive dietary advice (see Chapter 8).

Familial combined hyperlipidaemia
Originally, it was thought that there was a dominantly inherited hyperlipidaemia closely associated with CHD, but differing from FH.

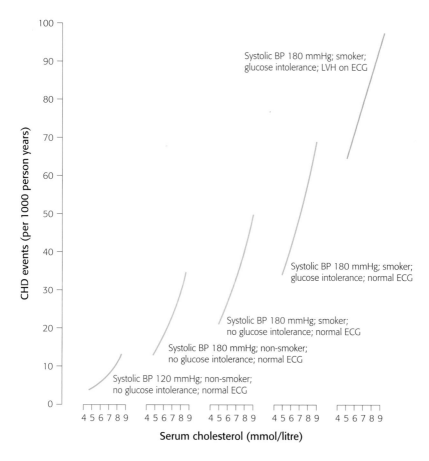

Figure 4.2 Coronary risk as a function of serum cholesterol and risk factors. ECG = electrocardiogram; LVH = left ventricular hypertrophy. Data from Anderson *et al. Am Heart J* 1990;121:293–8.

The lipoprotein phenotype within the same family could, with equal frequency, be a combined increase in cholesterol and triglycerides, an increase in triglycerides only or an increase in cholesterol only, and the disorder was called familial combined hyperlipidaemia. Affected families were thought to be about ten times more common than those with FH.

Subsequent research has not supported the concept of dominant inheritance. It appears that affected families have a type of polygenic

43

hyperlipidaemia, causing variable phenotypes among family members. Other features accompany combined hyperlipidaemia, and these are not seen with the more common type of polygenic hypercholesterolaemia. These include insulin resistance, or indeed frank diabetes, and hypertension. Furthermore, the serum HDL cholesterol is often low in affected members. Such families often come to medical attention because they manifest premature CHD. They appear to be at much greater risk than their serum cholesterol alone would indicate. It is not known with certainty whether this is because there are other, as yet undefined, genetic or acquired risk factors also running in these families, such as insulin resistance, or whether the nature of the dyslipidaemia itself is the reason for the increased risk. However, when estimating CHD risk (see Figure 10.1, pages 98–99), it is important to realize that family history can influence risk independently of the risk factors included in the calculation of risk. The true risk may therefore be greater than that estimated without inclusion of family history. Family history is also omitted from most other methods of estimating CHD risk.

Patients with hypertriglyceridaemia are at greater risk of CHD than are patients with similar cholesterol levels who do not have raised triglycerides. Hypertriglyceridaemia is, however, closely associated with a decrease in serum HDL cholesterol concentration, which is a stronger predictor of CHD risk in a multivariate analysis than serum triglyceride. This is because triglyceride values show greater variation, even when fasting, than do HDL cholesterol levels. It is now realized that serum triglycerides can profoundly affect the atherogenicity of LDL and, in many cases, are also the cause of the low HDL cholesterol. Furthermore, there is clinical trial evidence that lowering serum triglycerides in patients with a combined increase in both triglycerides and cholesterol decreases CHD risk. Similar evidence does not exist for raising HDL cholesterol. Therefore, in the treatment of hyper-lipidaemia to prevent CHD, triglycerides may be the next target after LDL cholesterol has been satisfactorily lowered.

Mechanism

Both polygenic hypercholesterolaemia and familial combined hyper-lipidaemia are associated with increased secretion of VLDL particles by the liver. Because VLDL is the precursor of LDL, this leads to increased LDL production. In many individuals, the LDL-receptor mechanism then becomes overloaded; the build-up of cholesterol is therefore due to the inability of LDL catabolism to cope in the face of increased LDL production without there being a rise in serum cholesterol concentration.

Raised LDL cholesterol/normal triglycerides. How is it that an increase in hepatic VLDL secretion can lead to an isolated increase in serum LDL cholesterol without there also being an increase in serum triglycerides? Serum triglycerides will generally increase only if VLDL rich in triglycerides accumulates in the plasma. In polygenic hypercholesterolaemia, the VLDL and hence triglyceride levels do not increase, despite the increased VLDL secretion, because VLDL is rapidly converted to LDL; furthermore, it may contain relatively fewer triglycerides and more cholesterol when it is secreted by the liver. In individuals who cannot rapidly convert the overproduced VLDL to LDL, combined hyperlipidaemia results. Indeed, some families with familial combined hyperlipidaemia seem to have a mutation of one of their lipoprotein lipase genes.

Apo B. Each VLDL particle has one molecule of apo B; this remains in the particle during its conversion to LDL and eventual catabolism. The serum concentration of apo B thus reflects the number of particles of VLDL and LDL in the circulation. Generally, at least 90% of serum apo B is present in LDL, reflecting the relatively high number of LDL particles in the circulation compared with VLDL particles. Both polygenic hypercholesterolaemia and familial combined hyperlipidaemia are therefore disorders of increased serum apo B or hyperapobetalipoproteinaemia.

Although both polygenic and familial combined hypercholesterolaemias have overproduction of VLDL and hyperapobetalipoproteinaemia in common, it has become increasingly evident that there is considerable individual variation in the degree of hypercholesterolaemia required to produce a given increase in serum apo B (Figure 4.3). Indeed, hyperapo-betalipoproteinaemia may be present in patients with no increase in serum cholesterol, such as those with pure hypertriglyceridaemia or occasionally people with apparently no increase in cholesterol or triglycerides. The explanation for this is that, whereas each LDL particle must contain one apo B molecule, it can vary greatly in the amount of cholesterol that it contains. Thus some people whose LDL is relatively depleted of cholesterol

45

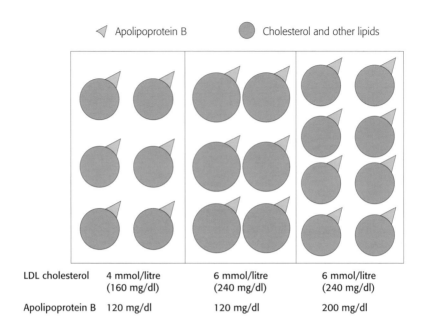

LDL cholesterol	4 mmol/litre (160 mg/dl)	6 mmol/litre (240 mg/dl)	6 mmol/litre (240 mg/dl)
Apolipoprotein B	120 mg/dl	120 mg/dl	200 mg/dl

Figure 4.3 The concentration of LDL particles in the serum is reflected in the serum apo B content, but because the quantity of cholesterol in each LDL particle can vary greatly from individual to individual, cholesterol concentration can be a poor guide to the LDL particle concentration.

can have an abnormally high LDL concentration without this being reflected in their serum cholesterol concentration – it will be evident only if serum apo B is measured. This may be important because the cholesterol-depleted LDL particles, which are also called small, dense LDL, are commonly associated with CHD and are often present in patients with hypertriglyceridaemia and insulin-resistance syndrome or diabetes.

Small, dense LDL. The explanation for the formation of small, dense LDL (and thus a higher circulating apo B level than would be anticipated from the serum or LDL cholesterol values) is that cholesteryl ester and triglycerides can exchange between the plasma lipoproteins, whereas the apo B present in LDL and VLDL cannot. The transfer of cholesteryl ester and triglycerides is mediated by CETP. This enzyme allows the transfer of cholesteryl ester from HDL and from LDL to the VLDL; the rate of transfer is increased when plasma VLDL levels are increased, as is typically the case in hypertriglyceridaemia. This leads to a decrease in HDL cholesterol and the formation of cholesteryl ester-depleted LDL.

Triglyceride moves from VLDL into both HDL and LDL. The triglyceride in LDL is, however, removed from LDL by a lipase enzyme present in the hepatic sinusoids. Thus, as the LDL passes through the liver, its triglyceride is removed. If it is already depleted of cholesteryl ester, this will create a smaller, denser particle. These particles are not taken up readily by the LDL receptor and are therefore removed more slowly from the circulation. They are more susceptible to oxidation than larger LDL particles and oxidized particles can be taken up by monocyte-macrophages in the arterial wall, leading to atheroma.

Because the LDL is depleted of cholesterol, measurements of serum or LDL cholesterol will not reveal the presence of the increased serum concentration of this type of LDL, though the LDL particle concentration may be high. This can be detected by measurement of serum apo B, but most laboratories do not perform this, so hyperapobetalipoproteinaemia may not be recognized. This probably accounts for patients who develop CHD prematurely without apparently having an elevated serum cholesterol concentration. Such patients often have some degree of hyper-triglyceridaemia and a low HDL cholesterol as the result of increased transfer of cholesterol from HDL to the triglyceride-rich lipoproteins. Clinically, therefore, patients with low serum HDL cholesterol, particularly when there is at least some degree of hypertriglyceridaemia, should be viewed with caution even when serum or LDL cholesterol is relatively normal.

Role of diet. Obesity and a high-fat diet (particularly one high in saturated fat) are probably the major reasons for the enormous differences in the prevalence of polygenic hypercholesterolaemia worldwide. Undoubtedly, however, individual responses to diet vary tremendously and there is probably a complex interplay between dietetic and genetic factors in the genesis of polygenic hypercholesterolaemia.

There is an impression that dietary modification aimed at lowering cholesterol in middle age in societies in which serum cholesterol is high does not reduce it to the extent that might be anticipated from populations habitually consuming such a diet. Whether this is simply a matter of non-compliance with diet or represents some permanent change in metabolism caused by a high-fat diet in early life is at present uncertain.

Physical signs in polygenic and familial combined hyperlipidaemias

Tendon xanthomata are absent in both disorders. Their presence in a patient with combined hyperlipidaemia indicates that the patient is one of the unusual patients with FH who have, in addition to increased LDL cholesterol, raised triglycerides, usually because they are obese. Obesity is generally not a prominent feature of FH, though it is common in polygenic and familial combined hyperlipidaemias. Xanthelasmata or corneal arcus occur in all types of hypercholesterolaemia regardless of aetiology. In patients with both hypertriglyceridaemia and hypercholesterolaemia, tubero-eruptive or striate palmar xanthomata generally indicate that the patient has type III hyperlipoproteinaemia (see Chapter 6); eruptive xanthomata are associated with severe hypertriglyceridaemia involving chylomicronaemia (see page 53).

CHAPTER 5
Hypertriglyceridaemia

Treatment is necessary to avoid the risk of acute pancreatitis in extreme hypertriglyceridaemia. The association of hypertriglyceridaemia with CHD is, however, complex and CHD risk is not necessarily dependent on the triglyceride level. This chapter examines patients with moderate hyper-triglyceridaemia, from 2.3 to 10 mmol/litre (200–900 mg/dl), and those with higher levels separately. There is no sharp division between these groups, however. Some people with apparently moderate-fasting hyper-triglyceridaemia have the capacity, under certain circumstances, to develop gross hypertriglyceridaemia leading to acute pancreatitis; others who habitually have serum triglyceride values of more than 30 mmol/litre (2700 mg/dl) can live to a ripe old age without complications.

Moderate hypertriglyceridaemia

The upper limit for fasting serum triglycerides is generally quoted as 2.3 mmol/litre (200 mg/dl), though the 95th percentiles for UK and US populations are closer to 3 mmol/litre (270 mg/dl). In univariate analyses of epidemiological studies, serum triglycerides are often stronger predictors of CHD risk than serum cholesterol. There is, however, a strong inverse relationship between serum triglycerides and the HDL cholesterol concentrations. The inclusion of HDL cholesterol in risk prediction substantially eliminates the effect of triglycerides on risk, though in meta-analyses of epidemiological studies, triglycerides still confer some independent risk even after taking HDL cholesterol into account.

A risk factor that apparently contributes little to CHD risk in multivariate analysis may be valuable clinically – multivariate analysis does not necessarily tell us which factors would be best corrected in order to prevent atheroma. Obesity, for example, does not emerge as an independent risk factor for CHD in multivariate analysis, unlike cholesterol, low HDL cholesterol, high blood pressure and diabetes mellitus. It would, however, be quite wrong to conclude that preventing or correcting obesity would not decrease CHD risk because, of course, obesity is a potent cause of hypercholesterolaemia, low HDL, hypertension and diabetes.

49

Drug treatment. There is no evidence that therapy aimed at decreasing serum triglycerides in patients whose serum cholesterol is below 5.0 mmol/litre (200 mg/dl) is of benefit in CHD primary prevention, although it may be justified in patients with established CHD. In patients without overt CHD whose serum cholesterol is above this level, the decision to treat with a lipid-lowering drug will depend on the patient's CHD risk. Generally this should be greater than 20% over the next 10 years (see Figure 10.1, pages 98–99). Before making the decision to introduce lipid-lowering drugs in patients with hypertriglyceridaemia, secondary causes should be sought and dietary advice given. In particular, excess alcohol consumption, liver disease, diabetes mellitus and renal disease should be excluded. Most of the patients with hypertriglyceridaemia considered for drug treatment will have a combined increase in cholesterol and triglycerides (type IIb hyperlipoproteinaemia or combined hyperlipidaemia).

Statins. When serum triglycerides are only moderately elevated, up to say 5.0 mmol/litre (450 mg/dl), a statin may be the best first-line treatment, because in addition to its cholesterol-lowering effect, it also decreases triglycerides and there is strong evidence that statins prevent CHD, generally without adverse effects (which is not known with the same degree of certainty for some other lipid-lowering drugs).

For patients whose hypertriglyceridaemia is too severe to respond to statin drugs, fish oil, fibrates and nicotinic acid should be considered.

Fish oil combined with a statin often decreases triglyceride levels satisfactorily. Fish oil has no cholesterol-decreasing effect. Although there is evidence that fish oil decreases CHD risk, this is not as strong as in the case of statins. It should not, therefore, be used alone.

Fibrates can be used as sole therapies, though their cholesterol-lowering effect is seldom adequate to achieve therapeutic targets for LDL cholesterol levels in, for example, myocardial infarction survivors. Indeed, in some patients with relatively low LDL cholesterol levels, these may initially increase on fibrate therapy.

Nicotinic acid is particularly effective at lowering both triglyceride and cholesterol levels. However, daily doses of several grams are generally required and at this level nicotinic acid has many side-effects (see Chapter 10).

Diet. Obesity is common in all types of hypertriglyceridaemia, in which case dietary advice should be directed at weight reduction. In those who are not overweight, or who fail to lose weight, generally restricting saturated fats is more effective than advice to restrict carbohydrate intake. Restriction of refined carbohydrate is, however, sensible.

In order to lose weight, decreases in overall fat intake may be required. In the case of severe hypertriglyceridaemia, when the contribution of chylomicrons is significant, a restriction in all types of fat intake is essential. Under these circumstances, carbohydrate intake may have to be increased in lean patients. Many patients with hypertriglyceridaemia are overtly diabetic. Others are glucose intolerant or will become so over the next few years. Weight reduction and dietary fat restriction improve glucose tolerance more effectively than carbohydrate restriction, because both measures decrease insulin resistance. It is insulin resistance that is generally the cause of diabetes or glucose intolerance in hypertriglyceridaemia, particularly when associated with CHD.

Effect of β-blockers. The indications for β-blockers should be reviewed, particularly if the hypertriglyceridaemia is marked. If β-blockers are clearly indicated, such as in patients with established CHD, bear in mind that we do not yet know whether minor elevations of triglycerides produced by β-blockers are harmful and thus whether any form of treatment is required. Marked elevation of triglycerides should be treated, however, in patients who cannot discontinue β-blockers.

Severe hypertriglyceridaemia (types I and V)
Diagnosis and underlying mechanism. In any circumstance that serum triglycerides exceed 10 mmol/litre (900 mg/dl), chylomicrons will be major contributors to the hyperlipidaemia, even when the patient is fasting. Chylomicrons and VLDL compete for the same clearance mechanism in the circulation (lipoprotein lipase). The lipoprotein phenotype is usually type V. This severe hypertriglyceridaemia generally occurs when an increase in hepatic VLDL production, either familial or secondary to, for example, obesity, diabetes, alcohol abuse or oestrogen administration, is associated with decreased triglyceride clearance. This again may be genetic or acquired, for example, in hypothyroidism, β-blockade or diabetes mellitus (diabetes

can cause both an overproduction of VLDL and decreased lipoprotein lipase activity).

With the clearance mechanism already overloaded with VLDL, the rise in serum triglyceride levels when chylomicrons enter the circulation following a fatty meal may be tumultuous and they may spend days rather than hours in the circulation. The serum takes on the appearance of milk (Figure 5.1) and triglyceride levels may exceed 100 mmol/litre (9000 mg/dl). A patient who might otherwise have a fasting serum triglyceride level of 5.0 mmol/litre (450 mg/dl) can, with the injudicious use of alcohol or the development of diabetes, achieve extraordinarily high serum triglyceride levels. Overall, the frequency of severe hypertriglyceridaemia is probably no more than 1 in 1000 in adults, and lower in children.

Familial lipoprotein lipase deficiency. Rarely, severe hypertriglyceridaemia is caused by familial lipoprotein lipase deficiency, a genetic deficiency in lipoprotein lipase activity. This is inherited as an autosomal recessive trait. It is usually due to mutation in the lipoprotein lipase gene, leading to defective function or production of the enzyme, but occasionally it results from a genetic deficiency of apo CII, the activator of lipoprotein lipase.

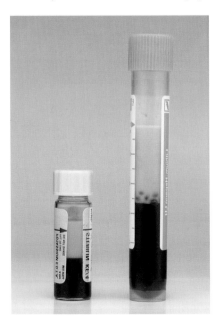

Figure 5.1 Milky serum in a patient with severe (type V) hyperlipoproteinaemia.

Severe hypertriglyceridaemia may present during childhood. Occasionally in children and young adults, familial lipoprotein lipase deficiency produces type I hyper-lipoproteinaemia, in which only serum chylomicron levels are elevated. It is not known for certain why the VLDL is not also raised, but it is likely that hepatic lipase can catabolize the lower levels of VLDL produced in childhood,

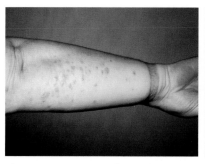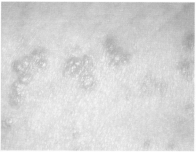

Figure 5.2 Eruptive xanthomata in a patient with severe (type V) hyperlipoproteinaemia.

although it is unable to compensate for the absence of lipoprotein lipase as far as chylomicron catabolism is concerned. With advancing age, VLDL production increases to levels above those that can be cleared by hepatic lipase. As a result, VLDL and chylomicrons accumulate in the circulation and type V hyperlipoproteinaemia becomes apparent.

Physical signs. Eruptive xanthomata are characteristic of extreme hypertriglyceridaemia. They appear as yellow papules on the extensor surfaces of the arms and legs, buttocks and back (Figure 5.2). Hepatosplenomegaly is common, and imaging shows the liver to be fatty. Bone-marrow biopsy may reveal foam cells. Because the triglyceride-rich lipoprotein may interfere with the determination of transaminases, giving spuriously high values, liver disease, in particular alcoholic liver disease, may be difficult to exclude other than by the prompt resolution of the syndrome when a low-fat diet is instituted. Other features include lipaemia retinalis, with both the retinal veins and arteries appearing white (Figure 5.3).

Atheroma is not a complication of familial lipoprotein lipase deficiency, but it does complicate severe hypertriglyceridaemia in which there is lipoprotein lipase activity, albeit diminished. It is difficult to make a precise estimate of the risk from the hyperlipidaemia because it is so commonly associated with insulin resistance or frank diabetes, which are themselves risk factors for atherosclerosis. If these are included as part of the syndrome, both CHD and peripheral arterial disease are common.

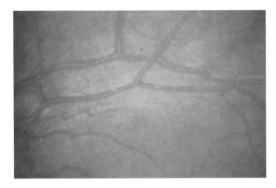

Figure 5.3 Lipaemia retinalis. Reproduced courtesy of Dr JP Miller, University Hospital of South Manchester, UK.

The reason that the complete absence of lipoprotein lipase removes the risk of atheroma is not known with certainty. It may be because:

- the incidence of diabetes is not increased in familial lipoprotein lipase deficiency
- fibrinogen and factor VII activity are not increased
- the conversion of VLDL and chylomicrons to the atherogenic intermediate-density lipoprotein (IDL) and remnant lipoproteins, respectively, is impaired in the absence of lipoprotein lipase
- serum LDL and apo B levels are often normal or decreased in familial lipoprotein lipase deficiency, any increase in serum cholesterol being due to the cholesterol in VLDL and chylomicrons.

Acute pancreatitis may occur when serum triglyceride levels exceed 20–30 mmol/litre (2000–3000 mg/dl). The presentation of acute pancreatitis is similar to that arising from other causes. However, increased serum amylase activity may not be present. Falsely low values may result from interference by triglyceride-rich lipoproteins in the laboratory method. All laboratories should inspect serum for milkiness (see Figure 5.1) before reporting normal or only moderately raised serum amylase activity in patients with severe abdominal pain. Clinicians may otherwise wrongly exclude the diagnosis of acute pancreatitis in favour, for example, of perforated peptic ulcer. Some patients do not develop acute pancreatitis, even when serum triglyceride levels exceed 100 mmol/litre (9000 mg/dl). Others may experience recurring acute episodes.

Chronic pancreatitis does not occur – generally the pain subsides within a few hours or days of starting nasogastric aspiration and intravenous fluids (with nothing being taken by mouth). Pseudocysts develop occasionally if treatment is delayed.

Recurrent abdominal pain, not typical of pancreatitis, sometimes occurs in patients prone to marked hypertriglyceridaemia. It may mimic irritable bowel syndrome. Severe abdominal pain may also be the result of splenic infarction.

Pseudohyponatraemia is another complication of extreme hyper-triglyceridaemia, and may lead to serious consequences if unrecognized. In pseudohyponatraemia, spuriously low serum sodium values are reported because much of the volume of the serum aliquot on which the sodium measurement is made is occupied by lipoproteins rather than water. When the serum triglycerides exceed 40–50 mmol/litre (3500–4500 mg/dl), the concentration of sodium in the aqueous phase (and thus the serum osmolality) may be normal, while spurious serum sodium levels of 120–130 mmol/litre are reported. The hazard is that these will be misinterpreted by the clinician and a patient already seriously ill with pancreatitis, or occasionally uncontrolled diabetes, will be made more so by infusion of large volumes of isotonic saline or worse, hypertonic saline.

Focal neurological syndromes such as hemiparesis, memory loss and loss of mental concentration may complicate extreme hypertriglyceridaemia; ischaemia may result from a sluggish microcirculation caused by the high concentrations of chylomicrons in the blood. Paraesthesiae, particularly in the feet, may also be an occasional feature, even in the absence of diabetes. *Sicca syndrome and polyarthritis* have also been described, but undoubtedly the most common articular association is with *gout* (see page 73).

Dietary modification. For patients with serum triglyceride levels exceeding 10 mmol/litre (900 mg/dl), fat intake of any type must be limited; chylomicrons persisting in the fasting state will be contributing to the hypertriglyceridaemia and these are formed from any kind of dietary fat. For patients with hypertriglyceridaemia prone to pancreatitis or with eruptive xanthomata and hepatosplenomegaly, restriction of daily fat intake to 20 g or below may be necessary. Medium-chain triglycerides and fish oil are of no value in this situation. Carbohydrate and proteins must be substituted for fat in patients who are not obese. A dietitian attached to a specialized unit is usually best placed to give this type of advice and training.

Drug therapy is generally less effective than a low-fat diet in severe hypertriglyceridaemia. Fibrates or nicotinic acid can, however, be of value.

CHAPTER 6
Type III hyperlipoproteinaemia

Type III hyperlipoproteinaemia has several synonyms:
- broad β disease
- floating β disease
- dysbetalipoproteinaemia
- remnant removal disease.

It is rare, probably affecting less than 1 in 5000 people, and rarer still in premenopausal women and children. Type III hyperlipoproteinaemia has the distinction of being the first clinical syndrome to be associated with primary hyperlipoproteinaemia, and was described by Addison (who also described adrenal insufficiency and pernicious anaemia) and Gull (physician to Queen Victoria) in 1851.

The condition is due to the presence of increased amounts of chylomicron remnants and IDL (or partially metabolized VLDL), often collectively termed β-VLDL, in the circulation. This is the result of decreased clearance of these lipoproteins at the apo E (or hepatic remnant) receptor.

Type III hyperlipoproteinaemia undoubtedly causes accelerated atherosclerosis in the coronary, iliac, femoral and tibial arteries. Intermittent claudication occurs at least as frequently as CHD and the incidence of the latter is about the same as that in FH. In FH, peripheral arterial disease is uncommon relative to the frequency of CHD, indicating that the atherogenic process in the leg arteries is much more susceptible to the larger lipoprotein particles in type III hyperlipoproteinaemia than the smaller LDL particles in FH.

Underlying mechanism
Type III hyperlipoproteinaemia is generally an autosomal recessive condition with variable penetrance. A mutation or polymorphism of the apo E gene appears to occur in all cases, and this impairs the binding of apo E to its receptor. A polymorphism, apo E_2, in which cysteine is substituted for arginine at position 158 (Figure 6.1), is the most common irregularity. At least 90% of patients with type III hyperlipoproteinaemia are homozygous for apo E_2.

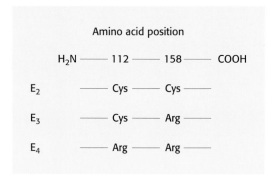

Figure 6.1 Amino-acid substitutions in the commonly occurring genetic polymorphisms of apo E.

More often than not, however, apo E_2 homozygosity, which is present in around 1% of the population, does not itself impose such a severe strain on lipoprotein metabolism that hyperlipoproteinaemia develops; its combination with some other disorder that causes overproduction of VLDL or some additional catabolic defect is required. This explains the association of type III hyperlipoproteinaemia with diabetes and hypothyroidism. More often, the additional stimulus to hyperlipoproteinaemia is obesity or the co-inheritance of a polygenic tendency to hypertriglyceridaemia. Rarer mutations of apo E have been described, including a mutation leading to apo E deficiency. These mutations behave similarly to apo E_2 homozygosity clinically, although they may not require other factors for the expression of the type III phenotype. Heterozygous apo E deficiency finds little clinical expression but, interestingly, mutations directly involving the receptor-binding domain of apo E (amino acids 124–150) produce the type III phenotype even in heterozygotes (dominant expression), implying that such mutations are a greater handicap to receptor clearance than mutations in which one gene does not produce apo E.

Diagnosis

Cholesterol and triglycerides. Serum cholesterol and fasting triglyceride concentrations are increased – typically 7–12 mmol/litre (270–470 mg/dl) for cholesterol and 5–20 mmol/litre (450–1800 mg/dl) for triglycerides. The molar concentrations of cholesterol and triglycerides are often similar, and this may be a clue that a patient has type III hyperlipoproteinaemia. Occasionally the condition is associated with marked hypertriglyceridaemia because of overwhelming chylomicronaemia.

Xanthomata are present in more than half of the patients with the type III lipoprotein phenotype. Striate palmar xanthomata (Figure 6.2) and tubero-eruptive xanthomata (Figure 6.3) are characteristic. Striate palmar xanthomata can simply be an orange discoloration of the palmar skin creases. They may, however, be more florid and appear as raised, seed-like lesions (sometimes even larger) in the skin creases of the palms, fingers and flexor surfaces of the wrists. Tubero-eruptive xanthomata occur over the elbows and knees, and sometimes over other tuberosities, such as the heels and dorsum of the interphalangeal joints of the fingers. They resolve entirely with successful treatment.

Laboratory tests. The diagnosis of type III hyperlipoproteinaemia is not difficult in the presence of typical xanthomata. When these are absent, laboratory tests are required. Type IIb or V hyperlipoproteinaemia can give similar serum lipid levels.

(a)

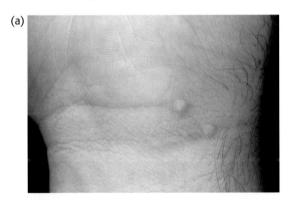

(b)

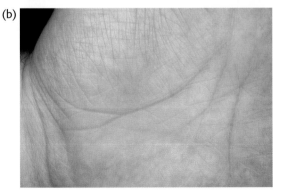

Figure 6.2 Striate palmar xanthomata (a) with some raised lesions, and (b) showing simply as an orange-yellow discoloration within the creases of the palm skin.

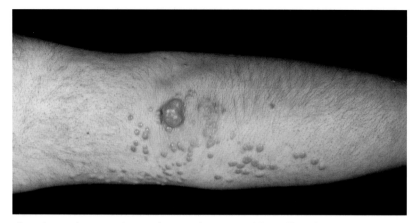

Figure 6.3 Tubero-eruptive xanthomata showing cauliflower-like tuberose on the point of the elbow and eruptive satellite lesions.

Lipoprotein electrophoresis is still available in some hospital laboratories and, when it clearly shows separate pre-β (VLDL) and β (LDL) bands, is useful in differentiating type IIb from III hyperlipoproteinaemia. Often, however, the classical broad β band associated with type III hyperlipoproteinaemia cannot be distinguished from the smear stretching from the origin into the pre-β and sometimes β regions in more severe cases of the IIb or type V phenotype.

Polyacrylamide gel isoelectric focusing or DNA testing by restriction-fragment-length polymorphism, available in many specialized centres, can be used to identify apo E_2 homozygosity. Apo E_2 homozygosity in the presence of hyperlipidaemia makes the diagnosis of type III virtually certain. When the apo E_2 homozygosity is absent in a patient with the typical type III clinical phenotype, some other apo E mutation is usually present. Its identification, though of great theoretical value at a specialized centre, is often impossible and, fortunately, of little practical importance.

Testing for the apo E genotype may reveal that a patient does not have type III hyperlipoproteinaemia, but provides the unwelcome finding that apo E_4 is present. This mutation has been linked with Alzheimer's disease – certainly in its late-onset form but also, in some studies, with the early-onset type. It is probably wise for the laboratory reporting the apo E genotype results to report only whether apo E_2 homozygosity is present or absent. Otherwise information about many people's apo E_4 genotype will be gratuitously available in their medical records without their consent or any explanation to them as to the possible consequences of its knowledge.

Ultracentrifugation. If clinical diagnosis of type III hyperlipoproteinaemia requires confirmation in the absence of apo E_2 homozygosity, plasma should be sent to a centre that can identify cholesterol-rich VLDL (β-VLDL) typical of type III using ultracentrifugation.

It is also important to exclude paraproteinaemia by immunoglobulin electrophoresis. This can produce hyperlipoproteinaemia mimicking type III.

Treatment

Diet. Type III hyperlipidaemia can be responsive to a reduction in obesity. In the occasional lean patient, a diet in which monounsaturated and poly-unsaturated fats and carbohydrates are substituted for saturated fat can be helpful unless triglycerides exceed 10 mmol/litre (900 mg/dl). If this is the case, a diet low in all types of fat, with carbohydrate substitution, may be necessary.

Fibrates. Type III is also generally responsive to fibrate drugs, which should be regarded as the first-line treatment option. If after dietary modification the triglycerides remain only moderately elevated and cholesterol is in the normal range, it is generally wise to introduce fibrate therapy, because even a moderate increase in triglycerides probably indicates that the abnormal β-VLDL is present in quantities that may still be harmful.

CHAPTER 7
Secondary hyperlipidaemia

Hyperlipidaemia commonly coexists with other diseases. These may occur as a complication of the hyperlipidaemia, as is the case with ischaemic heart disease in FH, and acute pancreatitis in marked hypertriglyceridaemia. Sometimes, however, a primary disease affects lipoprotein metabolism, increasing serum lipid concentrations. The resulting hyperlipidaemia is then properly regarded as a secondary hyperlipidaemia. Hyperlipidaemia may also be associated with another disorder more frequently than expected when neither occurs secondary to the other; the best example is hypertriglyceridaemia in gout, which is usually wrongly classified as a secondary hyperlipidaemia. It will, nonetheless, be considered in this chapter.

The secondary hyperlipidaemias are important because:

- the primary disease may be an important diagnosis in its own right
- the secondary hyperlipidaemia may be a cause of morbidity (e.g. ischaemic heart disease is now the major cause of premature mortality in diabetes and renal disease)
- disordered lipoprotein metabolism may accelerate the progress of the primary disease as has been suggested in renal and liver disease; lipoproteins probably have multiple functions besides that of lipid transport and their roles in cell membrane homeostasis and immunoregulation may be critical.

The secondary hyperlipidaemias (Table 7.1) are often associated not simply with increases in levels of circulating lipoproteins (Table 7.2), but also with changes in their composition, altering both their chemical and physical properties. This may influence the accuracy of laboratory methods developed for quantifying lipoproteins in primary hyperlipoproteinaemias. It may also mean that even when lipid levels are not clearly elevated, there may be qualitative changes in lipoproteins, perhaps rendering them more atherogenic. Dyslipidaemia or abnormal lipoprotein composition may eventually assume more importance than hyperlipidaemia in our understanding of atheroma, partly as a result of the study of secondary lipoprotein disorders.

TABLE 7.1

Diseases, physiological and pharmacological perturbations associated with secondary hyperlipidaemia

Endocrine

- Diabetes mellitus
- Thyroid disease
- Pituitary disease
- Pregnancy

Renal disease

- Nephrotic syndrome
- Chronic renal failure

Drugs

- β-blockers
- Thiazide diuretics
- Steroid hormones
- Microsomal enzyme inducing agents (e.g. phenytoin, phenobarbitone, griseofulvin)
- Retinoic acid derivatives (e.g. isotretinoin)

Hepatic disease

- Cholestasis
- Hepatocellular disease
- Cholelithiasis

Immunoglobulin excess

- Myeloma
- Macroglobulinaemia
- Systemic lupus erythematosus

Hyperuricaemia

Miscellaneous

- Glycogen storage disease
- Lipodystrophies

Nutritional

- Obesity
- Alcohol
- Anorexia nervosa

Diabetes mellitus

For too long, diabetologists have been guilty of regarding diabetes as simply a disorder of carbohydrate metabolism, and insulin as having the sole purpose of maintaining euglycaemia. The idea that diabetes is a disorder not only of carbohydrate metabolism, but also (and in many patients more importantly) of lipid and protein metabolism is slowly re-emerging. Two major complications of diabetes, atherosclerosis and ketoacidosis, are disorders of lipid metabolism and the possibility that there are others must never again be neglected.

TABLE 7.2

Effect of some secondary hyperlipidaemias on serum lipoprotein levels

Cause	VLDL	LDL	HDL
Type 1 diabetes	↑	– or ↓	– or ↑
Type 2 diabetes	↑↑	↑	↓
Hypothyroidism	↑	↑↑	↑
Pregnancy	↑	↑	↑
Obesity	↑	– or ↑	↓
Alcohol	↑	– or ↑	↑
Nephrotic syndrome	↑	↑↑	– or ↓
Chronic renal failure	↑	–	↓
Cholestasis	–	↑↑ (LpX)	↓
Hepatocellular disease	↑ (IDL)	–	↓
Hyperuricaemia	↑	–	↓

Hypertriglyceridaemia is the dominant hyperlipidaemia in diabetes mellitus. Lipoprotein lipase is activated by insulin. Thus insulin deficiency and/or resistance associated with uncontrolled diabetes may occasionally lead to spectacular elevations of serum triglycerides, sometimes to levels in excess of 100 mmol/litre (9000 mg/dl), and to the development of eruptive xanthomata and occasionally other features of the chylomicronaemia syndrome. Lipaemia retinalis can interfere with laser photocoagulation therapy for diabetic retinopathy. Those who develop this syndrome are probably genetically predisposed to hypertriglyceridaemia; generally a pre-existing partial defect in triglyceride catabolism exists. Sometimes tubero-eruptive xanthomata and striate palmar xanthomata indicate that florid type III hyperlipoproteinaemia has occurred in a genetically susceptible individual (usually an apo E_2 homozygote).

In most patients whose diabetes is under reasonable glycaemic control, any persisting hypertriglyceridaemia is not due to a major defect in triglyceride catabolism, but to overproduction of VLDL by the liver. NEFA arriving at the liver from the adipose tissue and skeletal muscle in increased quantities are likely to be a major reason for increased hepatic triglyceride synthesis. NEFA are released in increased quantities from adipose tissue when the quantity of adipose tissue is increased (i.e. obesity), which often occurs in non-insulin-dependent or Type 2 diabetes mellitus. Added to this, the enzyme within adipocytes that hydrolyses their stored triglyceride to produce glycerol and NEFA (hormone-sensitive lipase) is regulated by insulin. Insulin inhibits intracellular hormone-sensitive lipase, but activates lipoprotein lipase. Therefore, in insulin resistance, the hormone-sensitive lipase becomes active and NEFA are released from adipose tissue increases. At the same time, triglyceride clearance from the circulation may be diminished by the lowered activation of lipoprotein lipase.

In diabetes, triglyceride release from the liver is further facilitated by decreased insulin secretion and/or insulin resistance, which will decrease the direct inhibitory effect of insulin on the secretion of VLDL by hepatocytes. Even in insulin-treated diabetes, the liver is likely to remain deficient in insulin because insulin administered via the subcutaneous route arrives at the liver from the systemic circulation rather than via the portal vein; physiologically, the concentration of insulin in the portal circulation is several times that in the systemic circulation. To achieve such high portal insulin levels by systemic administration of insulin would subject peripheral tissues to grossly supraphysiological levels.

Patients with insulin-dependent or Type 1 diabetes mellitus tend to be less likely to have hypertriglyceridaemia than those with Type 2 diabetes. This may be partly because insulin therapy is the rule in Type 1 diabetes, and also because other factors predisposing to hypertriglyceridaemia, such as obesity, and β-blocker and diuretic therapies, are more common in Type 2 diabetes. There may, however, be a more fundamental reason. NEFA are disposed of by the liver in three major processes:

• complete oxidation
• partial oxidation (ketogenesis)
• esterification (triglyceride synthesis).

When hepatic energy requirements are met, only ketogenesis and esterification are possible. In Type 2 diabetes, NEFA are not readily converted to ketone bodies, whereas in Type 1 diabetes their entry into the mitochondria, where β-oxidation occurs, is facilitated for reasons not entirely understood. Resistance to ketogenesis in Type 2 diabetes may thus carry with it a predisposition to hypertriglyceridaemia.

Hypertriglyceridaemia is a much stronger marker for CHD in diabetic populations than in non-diabetic ones. Low HDL cholesterol levels often coexist with hypertriglyceridaemia, particularly in Type 2 diabetes. In patients destined to develop Type 2 diabetes, raised serum triglycerides and low HDL often precede the onset of glycaemia by many years. These patients yet to develop glycaemia of diabetic proportions will have insulin resistance. It is not certain to what extent the insulin-resistance syndrome is really pre-diabetes.

The atherogenicity of hypertriglyceridaemia in diabetes is unlikely to involve the triglyceride-rich lipoproteins responsible for the elevated serum triglyceride levels directly; it is likely to result from smaller apo B-rich lipoproteins produced by their catabolism. There is evidence that increased quantities of small LDL are produced in Type 2 diabetes with hypertriglyceridaemia. Also, in both types of diabetes, remnant particles or IDL probably persist at higher concentrations than in non-diabetics. There may also be a defect in the regulation of postprandial lipoprotein metabolism in diabetes. Normally the insulin secreted when the products of digestion enter the circulation inhibits hepatic VLDL secretion and promotes hepatic triglyceride storage at a time when triglyceride-rich lipoprotein production is high. This relieves pressure on the triglyceride catabolic pathways, such as those involving lipoprotein lipase and the apo E receptor, preventing the accumulation of remnants and IDL in the circulation postprandially. Later, when insulin levels decline, hepatic VLDL secretion increases and stored triglycerides are mobilized. In diabetes, failure to suppress VLDL secretion following meals occurs due to insulin resistance or deficiency, leading to high levels of remnant particles and IDL in the circulation.

Serum LDL cholesterol and apo B levels are, on average, somewhat increased in Type 2 diabetes populations compared with non-diabetic populations, whereas in Type 1 diabetes they are frequently normal or even a little lower. Potentially as important as the absolute levels of LDL is whether it is rendered more atherogenic (see Chapter 2). Recent evidence suggests that apo B, in addition to undergoing glycosylation, may be more subject to oxidative modification in diabetes. Collagen-advanced glycosylation end-products may also trap LDL in the arterial wall. Whatever the explanation, similar serum cholesterol levels in diabetic and non-diabetic people are associated with a greater coronary risk in those with diabetes. Many authorities now believe that after the age of 40, even in the absence of clinically overt vascular disease, serum cholesterol in diabetes should be treated as if the patient already had clinical CHD.

Serum HDL cholesterol concentrations tend to be low in Type 2 diabetes, whereas in Type 1 they are normal or even raised. The low levels in Type 2 diabetes are largely explained by the presence of associated hypertriglyceridaemia, obesity, cigarette smoking, abstemiousness from alcohol and the use of drugs such as β-blockers. These factors are less common in Type 1 diabetes and some other influence – probably insulin therapy – tends to increase HDL. A possible mechanism is that insulin increases HDL as a result of stimulating lipoprotein lipase activity.

Effect of drugs. Oral hypoglycaemic agents do not adversely affect lipoprotein levels in therapeutic trials, and improvements in glycaemic control may even produce some improvement in lipid profiles. Metformin and guar gum also probably have an independent lipid-lowering action. Sadly, the use of sulfonylurea drugs in clinical practice is linked with decreased HDL and probably other adverse effects, such as increases in triglycerides and cholesterol. This is because the use of these drugs in practice is all too often associated with body weight gain. Insulin too, though its action is to lower triglycerides and cholesterol and raise HDL, may stimulate weight gain and thus increase insulin resistance, which will tend to nullify or even reverse any beneficial effects.

Proteinuria, hypertension and hyperfibrinogenaemia often coexist with hyperlipidaemia in diabetes and increase coronary risk considerably. Nephropathy, as in the case of primary renal disease, may influence lipoprotein metabolism. Proteinuria in diabetes indicates a generalized increase in vascular permeability, and thus macromolecules such as LDL may enter the arterial subintima at increased rates – an effect aided and abetted by hypertension.

Thyroid disease

Serum LDL cholesterol and, more rarely, serum triglycerides are raised in hypothyroidism. Receptor-mediated LDL catabolism is decreased; triglyceride catabolism and lipoprotein lipase activity may also be reduced. HDL levels also tend to be increased due to diminished transfer of cholesteryl ester to other lipoproteins. These effects may be reversible with thyroxine replacement therapy (Figure 7.1), which also restores biliary cholesterol excretion to normal where it was previously depressed.

Subclinical hypothyroidism (raised serum thyroid-stimulating hormone, TSH, but thyroxine in the normal range) probably influences serum LDL slightly. In one survey, raised serum TSH was detected in 20% of women over the age of 40 years with serum cholesterol exceeding 8.0 mmol/litre (310 mg/dl). Although only 5% were actually hypothyroid, findings such as these underline the importance of adequately excluding hyperthyroidism in people with hypercholesterolaemia beyond mid-life.

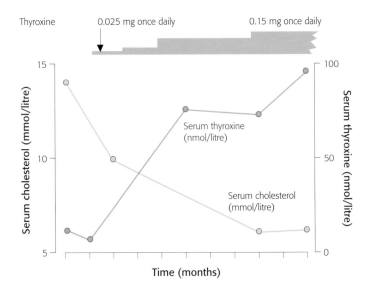

Figure 7.1 Effect of thyroxine-replacement therapy on serum cholesterol in a patient with hypothyroidism.

Hyperthyroidism. There is a tendency towards decreased LDL and HDL cholesterol in hyperthyroidism, but hypertriglyceridaemia can occur.

Obesity

Obesity will exacerbate any primary hyperlipoproteinaemia. Its dominant effect is to produce hypertriglyceridaemia, usually type IV hyperlipo-proteinaemia (occasionally type V), but in susceptible individuals, hypercholesterolaemia due to increased LDL will be exacerbated (type IIb). Android (male-pattern) obesity is more likely to provoke hypertriglyceridaemia than gynoid (female-pattern) obesity, assessed by determining the ratio of the hips to waist girth.

The cause of the hypertriglyceridaemia is increased hepatic VLDL production; this probably results from an increased release of NEFA from adipose tissue. This, in turn, stimulates hepatic triglyceride production. The increased VLDL secretion is sometimes matched by an enhanced catabolism due to increased lipoprotein lipase activity, so that hypertriglyceridaemia does not invariably ensue. Hypertriglyceridaemia is more likely if there is a pre-existing defect in triglyceride catabolism. Increased cholesterol synthesis also occurs in obesity, explaining why it can exacerbate hypercholesterolaemia.

Serum HDL cholesterol tends to be decreased in obesity. The explanation is uncertain, particularly when hypertriglyceridaemia is absent. Furthermore, whereas serum triglycerides and cholesterol decrease during weight reduction, there may be no increase in serum HDL cholesterol. Sometimes, if substantial weight loss is achieved and maintained, HDL does rise. However, patients able to achieve this degree of weight loss are a highly selected group and it is impossible to dissociate their weight loss from other lifestyle changes that might increase the serum HDL concentration.

Alcohol

Alcoholic beverages, particularly beer and wine, are energy rich and may be a cause of obesity. In addition, alcohol itself affects lipoprotein metabolism. Its dominant effect is to produce hypertriglyceridaemia by increasing hepatic triglyceride synthesis. In turn, this leads to increased VLDL secretion. Fatty liver ensues if the mechanism for VLDL assembly and secretion fails to keep pace with production of triglyceride. Usually, alcohol overindulgence produces type IV hyperlipoproteinaemia, but in individuals with a constitutional tendency to delayed triglyceride catabolism, a spectacular type V hyperlipoproteinaemia may occur; this may be one explanation for the association between alcohol consumption and acute pancreatitis. The increase in hepatic triglyceride synthesis stems partly from the ethanol-induced inhibition of oxidation of substrates other than itself. This tends to divert NEFA away from oxidative pathways into triglyceride synthesis. Triglyceride synthesis is further accelerated by the increased serum NEFA released from adipose tissue when ethanol is taken during fasting, or by the increase in food-induced fatty acidaemia induced by alcohol taken during a meal.

Serum LDL cholesterol levels tend to be low and HDL cholesterol raised in chronic alcoholics, unless liver disease has developed. The effect on HDL is evident in moderate drinkers, due predominantly to an effect on smaller HDL particles (HDL_3), whereas in heavy drinkers the measurably greater increase in HDL is due to the larger HDL_2.

Recognizing occult alcoholism is obviously important, particularly in hypertriglyceridaemic patients prone to pancreatitis. Measuring serum γ-glutamyl transpeptidase is not always helpful in identifying patients who drink heavily, because it may be raised in patients with hypertriglyceridaemia unrelated to alcohol.

Renal disease

Nephrotic syndrome. When proteinuria occurs in patients with relatively normal creatinine clearance, the predominant effect is to increase LDL (either from increased production of VLDL or by an increase in the amount directly secreted by the liver), thus producing hypercholesterolaemia. The severity of the hypercholesterolaemia is often proportional to the decrease in serum albumin.

Hypertriglyceridaemia in nephrotic syndrome is unusual in the absence of hypercholesterolaemia; it is more likely where chronic renal failure is also present, when it is often associated with decreased lipoprotein lipase activity. VLDL secretion by cultured hepatocytes decreases in response to albumin in the culture medium; the intravenous infusion of albumin or other macromolecules into patients with nephrotic syndrome reduces LDL levels. Both effects may be due to changes in osmotic pressure or to viscosity, as other macromolecules affect VLDL secretion in a similar way.

Serum HDL cholesterol levels are usually normal or decreased in nephrotic syndrome. Even when total HDL is normal, there is a shift towards smaller sized particles so that the HDL_2 subfraction decreases while HDL_3 often increases. Loss of HDL from the circulation increases because of leakage from the kidney, and this is related to the selectivity and extent of the glomerular leak. Immunoreactive apolipoprotein AI in quantities equal to the normal daily apolipoprotein AI production may be found in the urine; to maintain relatively normal serum HDL cholesterol levels, HDL production is greatly increased in many patients with proteinuria.

Chronic renal failure without proteinaemia. The proportions of serum triglycerides are raised in both VLDL and LDL in patients with renal failure. There is also a tendency for remnant particles to persist in the circulation. The underlying cause is uncertain, but may relate to decreased activity of both lipoprotein lipase and hepatic lipase. Insulin resistance associated with renal failure does not appear to increase NEFA flux as it often does in other conditions. Haemodialysis further exacerbates hypertriglyceridaemia; heparin depletes lipoprotein lipase and, in addition, there is loss of apolipoprotein CII, the activator of lipoprotein lipase, from the circulation. Chronic ambulatory peritoneal dialysis leads to the absorption of considerable amounts of glucose from the peritoneum, producing obesity and exacerbating hypertriglyceridaemia. In addition, LDL apo B is often raised, even when LDL cholesterol levels are not.

Serum HDL cholesterol levels are low in patients with chronic renal failure, while serum levels of lipoprotein (a) (Lp(a)) are often markedly elevated in all types of renal disease. Lp(a) comprises an LDL-like particle that contains apo (a) in addition to the usual apo B. Apo (a) is a member of the plasminogen supergene family and has much structural similarity with plasminogen. It appears to be an independent risk factor for CHD and cerebrovascular disease when it is present in high concentrations. Whether increased Lp(a) contributes to heightened susceptibility to atherosclerosis in renal disease is currently uncertain.

If good renal function is established, many of the lipoprotein abnormalities resolve following renal transplantation. However, hyper-lipidaemia persists in about one-quarter of patients, perhaps because of corticosteroid therapy, weight gain, antihypertensive therapy and, possibly, cyclosporin treatment.

Liver disease

Cholestasis. Hypercholesterolaemia occurs in obstructive jaundice without severe hepatocellular dysfunction. This is due to an increase in unesterified cholesterol in particles of hydrated density similar to that of LDL. Moderate hypertriglyceridaemia and an increase in the plasma phospholipid, lecithin (phosphatidylcholine), may also occur.

The lipoproteins of density similar to LDL are not true apo B-containing LDL, levels of which may be low, but are predominantly another lipoprotein designated lipoprotein X (LpX). This contains unesterified cholesterol and phospholipid in an approximately equal molar ratio. LpX has a lamellar structure and on electron microscopy appears as stacks of disc-like vesicles. LpX comprises 6% protein, of which at least half is albumin enclosed within the vesicles. Apolipoproteins, particularly apolipoprotein C, are present on their surface. LpX migrates towards the cathode on electrophoresis on agar (but not agarose), which is unusual for a plasma lipoprotein. Biliary cholesterol does contribute to the cholesterol of LpX, but diversion of this from the obstructed biliary tree back into the circulation is, on its own, insufficient to explain the extent of hypercholesterolaemia occurring in many patients. LCAT deficiency (see page 15) also contributes to the accumulation of unesterified cholesterol, but again this is unlikely to be the sole cause of the hypercholesterolaemia, because only relatively small quantities of LpX are formed when LCAT activity is even more profoundly decreased in familial LCAT deficiency. In patients with biliary obstruction, LpX in the blood appears to be largely due to the reflux into the circulation of biliary phospholipids, which attract cholesterol out of cell membranes.

LpX is catabolized by the reticulo-endothelial system, including Kupffer cells. Although it is not itself taken up by the hepatocyte, it may interfere with hepatic uptake of chylomicron remnants. The emerging view is that a system may exist for the sequestration of remnants in the space of Disse before uptake by the hepatocyte; it is interesting to speculate that this may be a site of their interaction with LpX. This may explain the persistence of remnant-like lipoproteins in patients with obstructive jaundice.

Hepatocellular disease is often accompanied by moderate hyper-triglyceridaemia. This is due to triglyceride-rich lipoproteins with density in the VLDL and LDL range, but which have β-electrophoretic mobility, forming a broad β-band on electrophoresis. The HDL present also has β-mobility and, when isolated in the ultracentrifuge, consists predominantly of small particles. The accumulation of small HDL and the decrease in cholesteryl ester is secondary to LCAT deficiency and the lipoproteins intermediate between VLDL and LDL probably build up because of hepatic lipase deficiency and other damage to the remnant-removal mechanism.

Hyperuricaemia and gout

Hyperuricaemia is present in a high proportion (probably half or more) of men with hypertriglyceridaemia. As a result, gout commonly presents in patients with hypertriglyceridaemia, particularly when hyperuricaemia has been further 'precipitated' by thiazide diuretic administration. The reason for the association is not entirely clear, as it appears to be more common than might be explained by the frequent coincidence of factors, such as obesity and high alcohol consumption, with hypertriglyceridaemia.

Hypertriglyceridaemia and hyperuricaemia are not causally related, as lowering uric acid with allopurinol does not affect triglyceride levels; conversely, with two exceptions, lipid-lowering drug therapy does not alter the serum urate concentration. The two exceptions are nicotinic acid, which raises urate, and fenofibrate, which lowers it. The latter effect, however, is not mediated through the triglyceride-lowering action of fenofibrate, but through an independent uricosuric effect. Both urate and triglyceride levels may decrease on a weight-reducing diet, suggesting that they may both be epiphenomena of some underlying nutritional process. Dietary carbohydrate is suggested to be of importance. Dietary fructose, which is taken up almost exclusively by the liver, induces hypertriglyceridaemia and also increases urate levels, probably by diverting energy away from the hepatic urate-scavenging pathway into fructose phosphorylation.

Drugs

A large number of drugs in common use affect serum lipoprotein concentrations (Table 7.3). Those most commonly encountered in the lipid clinic are diuretics and β-blockers.

TABLE 7.3

Drugs affecting lipoprotein metabolism

Drug	VLDL	LDL	HDL
Thiazides	↑	↑	–
β-blockers without ISA	↑	–	↓
Oestrogens	↑	– or ↓*	↑
Progestogens	–	↑	↓
Androgens	↓	↑	↓
Glucocorticoids	– or ↑	↑	↑
Hepatic microsomal enzyme-inducing agents (e.g. phenobarbitone, rifampicin, griseofulvin)	–**	–†	↑
Retinoic acid derivatives (e.g. isotretinoin)	↑	–	–

ISA = intrinsic sympathomimetic activity

*Decreased LDL in postmenopausal women

**May be unsustained increase

Thiazide diuretics raise VLDL and LDL by mechanisms that have not been elucidated. Their effect is generally small, but it may be more substantial in diabetes, which they also exacerbate. Diuretics do not alter HDL levels.

β-blockers, regardless of cardioselectivity, tend to increase serum triglyceride concentrations by an effect on VLDL, and to decrease HDL cholesterol. There is no convincing evidence that they affect total cholesterol or LDL cholesterol. Their effect on serum triglycerides may be marked in patients with pre-existing hypertriglyceridaemia. A decrease in the clearance of triglyceride-rich lipoproteins appears to be the mechanism, perhaps resulting from a direct effect in reducing the activity of lipoprotein lipase or from diversion of blood flow away from the vascular bed of muscle, one site rich in the enzyme.

β-blockers with intrinsic sympathomimetic activity (ISA) have little or no effect on serum HDL and triglycerides. Of this class, pindolol has the highest ISA, but has found little favour as an antihypertensive and is unsuitable for the management of angina. Acebutolol and oxprenolol, with ISA about half that of pindolol, but about double those of other β-blockers, may be valuable in some patients with hypertriglyceridaemia when β-blocker therapy cannot be avoided. Labetalol, which combines α- and β-blocking activity, is reported to have little effect on serum lipoproteins.

Many reports suggest that α-blockers, calcium-channel antagonist vasodilators, direct-acting vasodilators and angiotensin-converting enzyme inhibitors are either without effect on serum lipoproteins or may even have apparently favourable effects, such as raising HDL cholesterol. There is, however, no evidence as yet that pharmacologically induced changes of this type significantly alter disease morbidity or mortality.

Oestrogens tend to raise the serum triglyceride level due to increased hepatic VLDL production. Occasionally their administration in women with pre-existing hypertriglyceridaemia has led to gross hyperchylomicronaemia and consequent acute pancreatitis. In most women, the increase in triglycerides is small. Paradoxically, improvement has been reported in women with type III hyperlipoproteinaemia, possibly because oestrogen induction of remnant receptors outweighs any deleterious effect of increased VLDL production.

Oestrogens also raise serum HDL concentrations and, in post-menopausal women, decrease serum LDL levels. Although their effects may therefore appear beneficial, this idea must be tempered with caution. First, because the opportunities to administer oestrogen preparations alone are few; generally only postmenopausal women who have undergone hysterectomy can be considered. Oestrogen must be combined with a progestogen for most women requiring it for contraception or as hormone-replacement therapy. The final balance of favourable and unfavourable effects on lipid metabolism in any individual will then depend on the preparation used. Second, oestrogens increase the risk of thromboembolism and, like other steroids, will have mineralocorticoid and glucocorticoid activity, thus increasing the tendency to hypertension and diabetes mellitus.

Androgens generally cause the opposite effects to those achieved with oestrogens: a decrease in serum HDL cholesterol and VLDL and an increase in LDL.

Progestogens increase LDL and decrease HDL – the strength of the effect depends on their androgenicity.

Many drugs other than those discussed above affect lipoprotein metabolism (e.g. retinoic acid derivatives used in dermatology). Also important, because of the high rate of atherosclerosis in recipients of renal transplants, are the corticosteroids and cyclosporin used as immunosuppressive agents. Of great theoretical interest are drugs and chemicals that induce hepatic cytochrome P450, because of an associated increase in serum HDL levels. Such drugs include phenytoin, phenobarbitone, rifampicin and griseofulvin. Chlorinated pesticides, such as lindane and DDT, have the same effect.

CHAPTER 8
Dietary treatment

Recent criticisms levelled at the effectiveness of dietary treatment mostly stem from overviews of the effect of diet on lowering serum cholesterol in clinical trials. There is no doubt that clinical trials of diet are difficult to design and execute. Nevertheless, in practice, some people achieve a worthwhile reduction in cholesterol with dietary advice and it is cheap to implement in comparison with drug treatment.

Diet can decrease both cholesterol and triglyceride levels and can significantly improve glycaemic control in diabetes, sometimes even rendering the patient non-diabetic. The overviews of trials in which CHD incidence was the outcome measure also show that CHD risk can be diminished with diet. The fear of those critical of dietary treatment is that it may be employed as a sole means of therapy in high-risk patients who might otherwise derive considerable benefit from drug therapy. Diet should therefore be regarded as an adjunct to lipid-lowering drug therapy in patients at high CHD risk, such as those with established CHD. It should be part of the general lifestyle advice given to lower risk patients for whom lipid-lowering drug therapy is not justified (see Chapter 9).

Failure of dietary modification to decrease cholesterol below some arbitrary level is not in itself an indication for lipid-lowering drug therapy; generally the need for drug therapy is determined by CHD risk. It is sometimes questioned whether it is worth bothering with diet in high-risk patients when the statins, for example, can produce a much more substantial decrease in serum cholesterol. The reason for continuing to advocate dietary advice is that the decrease in CHD incidence in many dietary trials was apparently greater than would have been anticipated from the decrease in serum cholesterol achieved in the trials. It seems, therefore, that there may be some additional beneficial effects that patients relying exclusively on pharmacological measures are denied. Not to emphasize diet in CHD prevention is to broadcast the wrong message to the public and to those responsible for determining nutritional policy.

Dietary advice should be offered to most people whose serum cholesterol exceeds 5.0 mmol/litre (200 mg/dl). General advice is probably of limited value, if the cholesterol is substantially higher or there is concern about CHD risk. Referral to a dietitian or to a nurse who has trained in dietary counselling is then generally advisable. If the patient does not do the cooking in the household, then whoever does should also be present on such a visit. The importance of such a referral is that a personal dietary history will be taken so that advice can be tailored to the patient's own dietary preferences.

There are two essential components to dietary prevention of CHD – weight loss and reduction of saturated fat intake.

Weight reduction

Obesity is clearly related to hypercholesterolaemia, hypertriglyceridaemia, low HDL cholesterol (Figure 8.1), high blood pressure, insulin resistance and

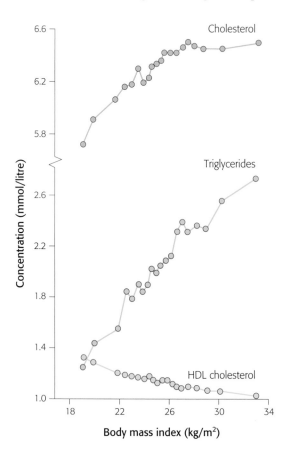

Figure 8.1 The effect of increasing degrees of obesity on serum lipids and HDL cholesterol. Reproduced with permission from BMJ Publishing Group from Thelle *et al. Br Heart J* 1983;49:205–13.

diabetes mellitus. The obese patient should be advised to lose weight. Even reduction of moderate obesity is sometimes helpful – all hyperlipidaemias in the obese respond to weight reduction. Failure to lose weight complicates the management of hyperlipidaemia, hypertension and diabetes. The best way to lose weight is to eat less, particularly fat. A consistent weight loss of about 1 lb/week (0.45 kg/week) is a very laudable target for weight reduction. Exercise cannot substitute for a reduced energy intake, except in unusual cases, but it may be critical in maintaining the decreased body weight achieved by dietary restriction. Claims that exercise alone can produce weight loss are generally based on calculations that neglect to subtract the energy expenditure of whatever else the patient would have been doing, had he or she not been exercising at the time.

Reducing saturated fat intake

The second important element of dietary modification involves decreasing saturated fat intake. Saturated fats in the diet increase both serum cholesterol and triglyceride levels; replacing them with carbohydrates (other than simple sugars and syrup), polyunsaturated fats or monounsaturated fats lowers the serum cholesterol and triglyceride levels. In the non-obese, in whom an energy deficit is not needed, a traditional north European and North American diet can be modified by:

- increasing the intake of potatoes, pulses, rice, pasta and fish
- using olive oil products, soya-bean, sunflower, safflower, corn or rapeseed oils.

Other dietary advice

Fruit and vegetables have a small effect in decreasing blood cholesterol in their own right because of their soluble fibre content. They can be eaten freely because they do not contribute to obesity and can enhance the variety of a healthy diet enormously. They may even protect against CHD in other ways, for example by providing antioxidants and folic acid.

Fibre. There is probably no point in deliberately advising the consumption of high-fibre foods, particularly those rich in insoluble fibre. Wheat bran has no effect on blood cholesterol and the so-called high-fibre diet has deterred many people from following a cholesterol-lowering diet.

Dietary cholesterol does not contribute greatly to blood cholesterol levels. It is probably wise to limit eggs to about three a week, but most patients can still enjoy avocado pears or shellfish when they get the chance. Foods are often labelled 'low in cholesterol'. This is unimportant. What is important is that they are 'low in saturated fat' if your patient is concerned with lowering blood cholesterol and 'low in fat' if the patient is mainly trying to lose weight. Refined carbohydrate, such as sugar in drinks and confectionery, should be avoided if the patient is trying to lose weight. The less-refined carbohydrate foods, such as bread, rice and pasta, beans and potatoes, have a much lower energy content than fat, and their consumption should be encouraged (in moderation only for those trying to lose weight).

Coffee. There is probably no point in restricting coffee intake as a means of lowering blood cholesterol, because its effect is small.

Alcohol is not harmful to the heart in moderate amounts. However, in the obese it may be a major source of excess energy intake. In hyperlipidaemia, particularly when associated with raised triglyceride levels, and in hypertension, it may be necessary to monitor a period of abstinence to assess the effects of alcohol.

CHAPTER 9
Drug treatment

It has become traditional to distinguish between secondary and primary prevention. Secondary prevention is therapy to diminish the progression and the complications of vascular disease in those with clinical manifestations, such as angina or myocardial infarction. Primary prevention aims to prevent the development of symptomatic disease in those who are asymptomatic. The two approaches are less different than they might seem. Given that participants in the trials of primary prevention conducted to date were middle aged or beyond, many would already have coronary lesions, although these would not be severe. Hence they had disease, but their status was beneath the horizon of the available diagnostic technology.

Lipid lowering to reduce the progression of coronary lesions (angiographic trials)

The earlier trials of both primary and secondary prevention were not encouraging, almost certainly because some of the trial designs were weak, but also, more importantly, because the pharmacological interventions then available were either ineffective, difficult to take, or both. The trial that changed the landscape of therapeutic possibility was the Familial Atherosclerosis Treatment Study (FATS), the first lipid-lowering trial carried out using quantitative coronary angiography. FATS demonstrated that marked lowering of LDL, whether produced by a statin plus cholestyramine or by nicotinic acid plus cholestyramine, significantly reduced the rate of progression of coronary lesions. Although it was not designed to test whether clinical events would also be reduced, there was, in fact, a significant reduction in these as well.

Although scepticism remained, the nihilistic logjam was broken, and a substantial number of angiographic trials, many of which used statin monotherapy, were completed relatively quickly. The results were strikingly similar. With a single exception, the trials showed that angiographic progression of coronary lesions was reduced. The rate at which new lesions appeared also diminished – an important observation given the frequency with which clinical events are due to the rupture of non-occlusive lipid-rich plaques.

Although the individual trials were relatively small, a number showed a reduction in clinical events; taken together, an impressive improvement in clinical outcome was evident, with infarction and death reduced by more than 25%. The interventions used in these trials included not only statins and fibrates used as monotherapy and combinations of niacin and resins or statin and resins, but also diet and exercise regimens. Outcomes correlated both with changes in triglycerides and LDL.

Secondary prevention trials

Overall results. In the past few years, several randomized, controlled, blinded clinical trials of LDL lowering with statins for the secondary prevention of CHD have been completed. A number have been fully reported, while only preliminary analyses of others are available at the time of press. Taken together, they provide incontestable evidence that LDL lowering will significantly reduce the risk of death and coronary events in most patients with symptomatic CHD.

The first of these landmark trials was the Scandinavian Simvastatin Survival Study (4S trial) in which simvastatin was administered to moderately hypercholesterolaemic patients with known CHD. Total mortality was significantly reduced, as was the rate of coronary events. The two other major trials of secondary prevention for which data are available are the Cholesterol and Recurrent Events (CARE) and the Long-term Intervention with Pravastatin in Ischaemic Disease (LIPID) trials, both of which used pravastatin. In CARE, the sum of fatal and non-fatal coronary events was significantly reduced, while in LIPID both total and coronary mortality rates were reduced in the treated group compared with the control. The results from the three trials are summarized in Figure 9.1.

The patients in the CARE and LIPID trials had total and LDL cholesterol levels that were lower than in 4S. In the CARE trial, all subjects had a total cholesterol below 6.2 mmol/litre (240 mg/dl) with the average being 5.4 mmol/litre (209 mg/dl). The average LDL cholesterol was reduced from 3.6 to 2.5 mmol/litre (139 to 98 mg/dl). Although overall benefit was shown in the treated group in CARE, subgroup analysis showed no significant improvement in outcome for the treated group starting with an LDL

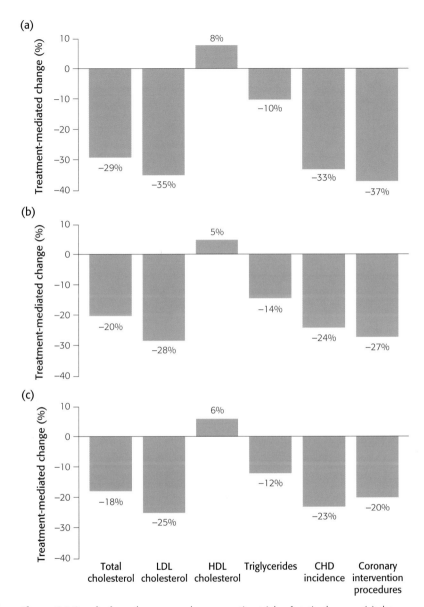

Figure 9.1 Results from three secondary prevention trials of statin therapy: (a) the Scandinavian Simvastatin Survival Study (4S), (b) Cholesterol Recurrent Events study and (c) the Long-term Intervention with Pravastatin in Ischaemic Heart Disease Study. The mean serum cholesterol values at randomization were 6.7 mmol/litre (260 mg/dl), 5.4 mmol/litre (209 mg/dl) and 5.6 mmol/litre (216 mg/dl), respectively.

cholesterol below 3.2 mmol/litre (125 mg/dl). Much attention has been paid to this finding, particularly when it is tied to findings in an earlier coronary angiographic trial, the Harvard Atherosclerosis Reversibility Project (HARP). If valid, it is of importance as it would argue against LDL lowering as secondary prevention in a substantial number of patients with coronary disease in countries such as the USA (though only a few in the UK where serum cholesterol levels are higher than in the USA). But the finding is far from definitive. It is a subgroup analysis and the number of subjects is too small for the result to be of high confidence.

The major argument against the CARE analysis lies in the results of LIPID, a larger trial with the same agent. In LIPID, there was no evidence of reduced benefit in those with lower cholesterol levels. Furthermore, HARP cannot be taken as strong confirmatory evidence, because it is contradicted by other similar trials. Thus, although it remains possible that there is a level below which LDL lowering is not of benefit, on the basis of the available evidence, we suggest it would be unreasonable to deny therapy arbitrarily on these grounds.

Subgroup results. Some subgroup analyses of 4S, CARE and LIPID are concordant and important.

Diabetic patients benefit in all three studies, the trend being positive but not statistically significant in LIPID, but achieving statistical significance in both CARE and 4S. Given the incidence of vascular disease in diabetes and the frequency of diabetes, this is potentially a major finding. It may be somewhat surprising as hypertriglyceridaemia and low HDL cholesterol are the features of diabetic dyslipidaemia that have been stressed, whereas the small, dense highly atherogenic LDL have been overlooked. Since the primary effect of the statins is to lower LDL particle number, these findings point to LDL being of major importance in the pathogenesis of atherosclerosis in diabetes. Other therapeutic options are being tested in diabetes, including fibrate therapy. The results are awaited with great interest and certainly a prospective trial of statin therapy in diabetes is essential before final conclusions are possible.

Women. That women benefit at least as much as men and perhaps more so is another critical subgroup finding. The effect of coronary disease on life expectancy is almost as great in women as it is of men, although onset is somewhat delayed. Clinical trials have not included as many women as they should, but on the basis of the available evidence there seems no reason to hesitate to treat women with coronary disease as vigorously as men.

Older patients. If there is no other obvious life-threatening or severely life-diminishing medical problem, those aged 65–75 years should obtain substantial benefit from therapy. Most coronary events occur in older people and therefore even moderate reductions in relative risk will produce marked gains in terms of the absolute number of events avoided.

Cerebrovascular accidents were significantly reduced both in CARE and LIPID, and there was a strong trend to benefit in 4S. A number of meta-analyses strengthen the results of the individual trials. There are, therefore, two arguments for LDL lowering in patients with cerebrovascular disease: first, there is a high likelihood of associated, even if asymptomatic, CHD in such patients and the coronary outcome will be improved with statin therapy. Second, the natural history of the cerebrovascular disease should be improved. As with diabetes, before the issue is considered finally settled, a trial committed to preventing vascular events in patients with cerebro-vascular disease (stroke or transient ischaemic attacks) would seem essential.

What do we still not know? A number of simple but critical clinical questions remain unresolved.

Definition of therapeutic targets. To date, the best-designed trials of secondary prevention have used statins, and lowering of total and LDL cholesterol have been the principal therapeutic targets. But to what level should they be lowered? The question is critical because it will define the extent of benefit possible from this therapeutic approach. At the moment, as achieved in the trials to date, moderate lowering of LDL cholesterol over the medium term will reduce overall death rates by about 25% and cardiac events by somewhat more. That means the majority of events will still occur and only the minority of patients will be helped. But would more intensive or more prolonged therapy produce greater benefit? Until clinical trials designed to answer this question have been completed, clinical judgement will continue to be required.

The target of therapy needs to be defined more precisely. In this evidence-based modern medical world, it should be noted that the American National Cholesterol Education Program (NCEP) target of an LDL cholesterol under

100 mg/dl (2.5 mmol/litre) appears to have been chosen arbitrarily. That is not to say that it will not, in time, be seen to be a reasonable judgement, but in the meantime, it remains an open question as to whether the target itself is correct. Whether we should aim for percentage reductions from levels on presentation rather than absolute levels also remains open.

Should other therapeutic targets be included? These might include triglycerides and HDL cholesterol. No definitive answers are available. The epidemiological evidence implicating both is strong. On the other hand, increased serum concentrations of small, dense LDL tend to be present in patients with CHD and hypertriglyceridaemia and low HDL cholesterol. Given that there are always many more LDL than VLDL particles, and given that smaller LDL particles are even more atherogenic than their normal-sized cousins, it seems easily possible that high triglycerides and low HDL cholesterol are markers pointing to the true villains of the piece – the small, dense LDL. Triglycerides may, however, be more than simple markers because there is increasing evidence that their presence leads to the generation of small, dense LDL and that lowering their concentration (e.g. with fibrates) decreases small, dense LDL concentration.

Our understanding of the pathogenesis of the risks of high triglycerides and low HDL cholesterol is currently incomplete. There are clinical trial data that indicate that reducing triglycerides could produce clinical benefit. The decrease in CHD incidence with fibrates is of a similar order of magnitude to that achieved with the statins, despite the much greater effect of statins on the larger cholesterol-rich LDL, reflected in their greater effect on serum cholesterol. For the moment, however, it seems premature to rate the effects of fibrates as being on a par with statin-mediated LDL lowering in coronary patients. Nevertheless, fibrate therapy may be justified in appropriate circumstances; for example, they could be used in combination with statins for patients with mixed hyperlipidaemia who are at particularly high risk (e.g. patients with established CHD and/or diabetes), as long as adequate monitoring to avoid myositis can be undertaken. Once more, we will have to fall back on clinical judgement for some considerable time yet.

Primary prevention trials

There are fewer data on primary prevention with statins. Two trials, the West of Scotland Coronary Prevention Study (WOSCOPS) and the Air Force/Texas Coronary Atherosclerosis Prevention Study (AFCAPS/TexCAPS), have been published to date (Figure 9.2). WOSCOPS involved middle-aged moderately hypercholesterolaemic men, many of whom were smokers. The trend to benefit was clear, with a significant reduction in the number of events though not quite in mortality. The degree of benefit in terms of relative risk reduction in AFCAPS/TexCAPS was

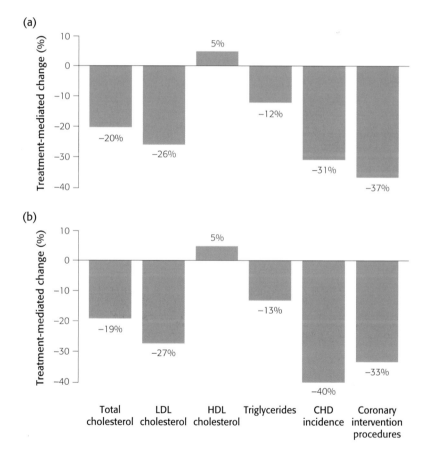

Figure 9.2 Results from the two primary prevention trials of statin therapy: (a) the West of Scotland Coronary Prevention Study (WOSCOPS), and (b) the Air Force/Texas Coronary Atherosclerosis Prevention Study (AFCAPS/TexCAPS). The mean serum cholesterol (TC) values at randomization were 7.0 mmol/litre (270 mg/dl) and 5.7 mmol/litre (220 mg/dl), respectively.

similar to that achieved in the secondary prevention statin trials. The major difference was in the absolute number of clinical events. The most important risk factor for a coronary event is the presence of coronary disease. Patients with coronary disease are overwhelmingly likely to die of it. Therefore, in trials of secondary prevention, there will be lots of coronary events to prevent.

The same is not the case for primary prevention, and one clear lesson from WOSCOPS and AFCAPS/TexCAPS is that lipid levels alone, except for those with extreme elevations, are relatively weak individual predictors of risk. Therefore, any prevention strategy either exclusively or primarily based on lipid levels will require a very large number of patients to be treated for any significant number to benefit. It is for this reason that calculation of absolute coronary risk is helpful in deciding who to treat in primary prevention.

A number of cost–benefit analyses have been published. Statin therapy is expensive, but the cost in relation to benefit diminishes as the risk of disease increases. In all these studies, yearly costs for treating one individual are usually favourably compared with standardized costs for individuals with other problems, such as end-stage renal disease requiring haemodialysis. However, it must be emphasized that cost–benefit studies must project total costs rather than just listing individual costs. The benefit of statin therapy clearly outweighs cost in secondary prevention, and in primary-prevention patients whose absolute CHD risk exceeds 20% in the next 10 years. As the cost of statins diminishes, lower levels of risk may justify treatment; they may already do so when treatment costs are borne by the patient. It should not be ignored that benefit was shown in AFCAPS/TexCAPS when CHD risk was only 1%, so the decision to employ statin therapy only in patients at higher risk is based not on scientific evaluation of the evidence, but on cost alone.

Guidelines

Generating national and multinational medical guidelines has become an enormous growth industry. These attempts at educating and advising physicians are important and necessary exercises. However, scientific rigour may occasionally play second fiddle to the necessity for consensus and, perhaps even worse, simplification by the expert for the non-expert.

Statements of the highest importance suddenly appear without any link to evidence. Nevertheless, there is an encouraging tendency, particularly apparent in recent guidelines such as those jointly agreed by the British Cardiac Society, British Hyperlipidaemia Association and British Hypertension Society, to take a more inclusive and balanced approach to risk-factor analysis, considering evidence in the widest context. This is crucial for primary prevention because plasma lipid values, except when extreme, are only crude and weak indicators of risk.

Hypertension, diabetes, smoking, male gender and family history are important risk factors. So is android obesity. Age becomes an ever more dominant risk factor as the decades pass. These risk factors may be thought of as either affecting LDL or affecting the interaction of LDL with the arterial wall as is discussed in Chapter 2. A relatively low level of LDL cholesterol may justify treatment in a patient with a particularly adverse combination of these other risk factors, whereas substantially higher levels of LDL cholesterol may not do so in the absence of these other risk factors. An important exception to this is FH, where the natural history of the condition dictates that statin treatment is generally started in men at least by their early twenties and women by their mid-thirties. More nebulous, but potentially important clinical syndromes, such as familial combined hyperlipidaemia, can also guide prognosis and treatment.

Pharmacotherapy

Diet almost always precedes pharmacological therapy in the advocated regimens. Unfortunately, dietary therapy is rarely more than partially successful and the reality for most individuals is that medication is required to achieve major changes in plasma lipoprotein levels. However impressive the safety record to date, lipid-lowering pharmacological therapy potentially carries some risk, which should never be overlooked. Moreover, the costs of therapy are substantial. They include not only the costs of the medication, but all the associated costs, such as laboratory, medical and nursing resources. But the costs go even further. There is loss of time from work to attend clinics and there is often an increase in absenteeism in those labelled with chronic medical diagnoses. That said, in those who can benefit, pharmacological therapy is well justified.

Statins inhibit HMG-CoA reductase (see page 8). Their principal effect is to lower plasma LDL, although modest increases in HDL cholesterol, and, depending on the agent and dose, variable decreases in plasma triglycerides also result. While LDL particle number and LDL cholesterol are substantially reduced, no changes in LDL particle composition result. Postprandial remnant clearance may also be improved in some patients.

By altering the balance of cholesterol and cholesteryl ester within the hepatocyte, statins increase the removal of IDL and LDL, and decrease the production of VLDL and LDL. Although a number of non-lipoprotein effects have been reported, such as a decrease in platelet aggregability and decreased smooth-muscle cell proliferation within the arterial wall, the effects on the plasma lipoproteins – in particular the marked decrease in LDL – would appear to be the major mechanisms underlying clinical benefit.

On the basis of the evidence from clinical and angiographic studies, statins should be regarded as first-line therapy for patients with atherosclerotic vascular disease. The currently available agents differ somewhat in their pharmacological properties and potency. Most often used as monotherapy, statins have been used in combination regimens when LDL levels are particularly high and sometimes when it is necessary to lower both LDL and triglycerides. Addition of bile-acid sequestrants will result in further lowering of LDL without any increase in the risk of side-effects. This combination can be unsuitable where a clinically significant increase in triglycerides as well as LDL cholesterol persists after statin therapy has been introduced, because hypertriglyceridaemia is often exacerbated by bile-acid sequestrating agents.

For this reason, notwithstanding the slight increase in the risk of toxicity, statins have also been combined with fibrates, particularly in patients with familial combined hyperlipidaemia, in order to reduce triglycerides more profoundly and to increase HDL cholesterol more markedly. This regimen will also alter LDL composition so that a smaller proportion of the more atherogenic small, dense LDL particles will persist. A newer combination therapy for combined hyperlipidaemia has been omega-3 fatty acids and statins – good results have been reported.

The statins currently available are atorvastatin, cerivastatin, fluvastatin, lovastatin, pravastatin and simvastatin. All are of proven efficacy in lowering LDL cholesterol, but so far, only lovastatin (not available in the UK), pravastatin and simvastatin have been shown in clinical trials to decrease CHD risk. Thus, if the clinician were to practice strictly evidence-based medicine, these drugs should be employed in the doses used in the trials with coronary events as end-points (that is, lovastatin 20–40 mg, pravastatin 40 mg and simvastatin 10–40 mg daily). To employ different doses of these drugs or to use the other statins is to extrapolate from clinical trials and to regard the coronary prevention action of the statins as a class effect. Although this may be attractive on the grounds of cost, such a view may be premature. In the case of atorvastatin, its use may be justified in patients with particularly high LDL levels, because it is the most effective of the statins, in terms of LDL lowering, in the doses that are currently available.

Side-effects. About 1% of patients have a substantial (more than three-fold), persistent but asymptomatic elevation of hepatic transaminase levels. The effect is usually dose related. Therapy may be continued in the face of mild increases in enzyme levels, although substantial increases call for discontinuation. Following normalization of hepatic function, re-institution of treatment at lower doses of a different statin should be considered. Hepatic enzyme levels should be measured 6 and 12 weeks after starting therapy, and semi-annually thereafter.

Asymptomatic elevation of creatine kinase, muscle weakness, pain or stiffness may occur. More rarely, frank rhabdomyolysis with acute renal failure will result, usually when statins have been given in combination with other hypolipidaemic agents, such as fibrates or nicotinic acid, or concurrently with agents such as cyclosporin in heart and renal transplant patients. The frequency of severe adverse reactions in these circumstances is happily much lower than was originally believed, and combination therapy may be used with caution in fully informed, frequently monitored patients. There is also a risk of myositis in patients on statin therapy when antibiotics such as erythromycin are administered. Such combinations should be avoided.

Levels of creatine kinase reaching two or three times the upper limit of laboratory reference ranges are not uncommon in patients not receiving lipid-lowering therapy. Sometimes these can be linked to bouts of muscular exertion. The clinician should be aware that such increases can occur spontaneously and are not necessarily the result of statin therapy. Furthermore, muscular ache, particularly in the shoulders and neck, is a common phenomenon that can lead to inappropriate discontinuation or rejection of statin therapy.

Although the evidence is incomplete, some experimental data suggest that statins have a teratogenic effect; administration during pregnancy, therefore, is inadvisable. On the other hand, there is no evidence of mutagenic effects.

As with any class of drugs, a range of side-effects such as headache, nausea, non-specific skeletomuscular symptoms and tiredness may be reported with statins. In placebo-controlled trials, these have not been reported with a substantially greater frequency in treated groups than in placebo groups. Nevertheless, they are the most commonly reported side-effects. Changing to another statin agent is often helpful.

Fibrates generally have a much weaker effect on LDL cholesterol levels than that of statins. Indeed, there may be an increase in LDL cholesterol concentration with these agents in patients with raised triglycerides and relatively low LDL cholesterol levels at the outset of treatment. They are effective in decreasing the circulating concentration of small, dense LDL, although the clinician is not in a position to assess this effect from routinely available lipid measurements.

The mechanism of action of fibrates is not well understood, but may include decreased triglyceride production by the liver and improved triglyceride clearance by peripheral tissues. The most important clinical effects are a marked reduction in serum triglycerides and an increase in HDL cholesterol. Depending on the agent and the type of hyperlipidaemia, LDL cholesterol and apo B levels may be reduced, but not usually by more than 10–20%. Postprandial triglyceride clearance is also improved after fibrate therapy.

Fibrates have been used in four major clinical trials: clofibrate in the Coronary Drug Project and the WHO Clofibrate Trial, and gemfibrozil in the Helsinki Heart Trial and the Veterans' Affairs High-Density Lipoprotein Cholesterol Intervention Trial. None showed a decrease in overall mortality, although CHD incidence was decreased. This may reflect trial design rather than clinical efficacy. Better designed, large clinical trials are currently underway. Bezafibrate and gemfibrozil have been shown to reduce angiographic progression of CHD.

Fibrates are certainly the pharmacological agents of choice in individuals with markedly elevated triglyceride levels and who are therefore at risk of pancreatitis. Normalization of plasma lipids also frequently occurs in patients with type III hyperlipoproteinaemia. In other patients with vascular disease, lack of trial data demonstrating clinical efficacy means statin therapy should be first-line therapy. It is possible that in subgroups such as those with diabetes, fibrates may bring particular benefit given the characteristic lipid profile of hypertriglyceridaemia, low HDL cholesterol and small, dense LDL in these patients, but again this awaits confirmation.

Side-effects are generally mild. Headache, gastrointestinal upset, rashes and pruritus have been reported. Mild elevations of hepatic and muscle enzymes may occur. Bile-acid lithogenicity is probably increased, at least in the early stages of treatment. Fibrates should be avoided in patients known to have gallstones, although only clofibrate has been shown in clinical trials to increase the incidence of clinically significant cholelithiasis.

Fibrates may interact significantly with anticoagulants such as warfarin, and great care should be exercised in their introduction in patients receiving such therapy. Their use should be avoided in patients with renal disease (bezafibrate, in particular, raises creatinine levels) and may cause a paradoxical rise in cholesterol in patients with cholestatic liver disease in whom they are contraindicated.

Bile-acid resins. The currently available agents are non-absorbable anion exchange resins that bind bile salts irreversibly. The resulting depletion in the bile-acid pool leads to greater breakdown of cholesterol to form bile acids. In turn, this leads to up-regulation of LDL receptors to maintain the cholesterol pool within the liver, and lowering of LDL levels typically by 10–20% (more in compliant patients). Plasma triglyceride levels, however, may increase substantially, particularly in those with already elevated values.

The major indication for these agents is in combination with a statin in patients with very high LDL levels. Under these circumstances, benefit can often be achieved with smaller, more acceptable daily doses (cholestyramine, 4–8 g; colestipol, 5–10 g). Stool softeners can be considered. There is an increased likelihood of gallstones developing with bile-acid sequestrants, although this may be lower in patients already receiving statins. Bile-acid sequestrants can decrease serum folate levels and folate supplementation

93

should be considered in vulnerable groups such as children and women who may become pregnant. In the Lipid Research Clinics Trial, cholestyramine decreased CHD incidence and both cholestyramine and colestipol have been used either alone or in combination with other drugs in successful coronary angiographic regression trials. Evidence that they significantly decrease all-cause mortality is not available, however, and it is unlikely that further trials will be undertaken to test this.

Side-effects. Constipation, bloating and heartburn are the principal side-effects and are commonly encountered, limiting the usefulness of this class.

Nicotinic acid is a B vitamin that, in pharmacological doses (up to 7 g daily), markedly reduces VLDL and LDL and substantially increases HDL. It alone among the hypolipidaemic agents may reduce Lp(a). Its mechanism of action is not certain, but involves reducing VLDL secretion by the liver, perhaps in response to reduced fatty acid release by adipocytes.

The advantages of nicotinic acid are that it improves the whole lipo-protein profile, and its cost is low. Opinions are divided about whether the dose should be taken all at once with the evening meal, allowing flushing (see below) to be endured in the privacy of one's own home, or whether it should be taken in divided doses to try to minimize side-effects. In either case, it is customary to begin with 50 mg daily, working up to a dose of 3000 mg or above. The dose should be taken at the end of a meal with a small dose of aspirin at the beginning. Lipoprotein levels should be assessed 1 month later.

Side-effects limit its use. Flushing is virtually universal. It can be reduced if a small dose of aspirin or another prostaglandin inhibitor is taken shortly before nicotinic acid. More serious side-effects include gastritis and peptic ulcer exacerbation, hepatitis, gout and hyperglycaemia. Significant inter-action with statins can occur to produce rhabdomyolysis and renal failure.

Analogues and slow-release preparations. Because of its attractive effect on the lipoprotein profile, numerous attempts have been made to produce analogues or preparations of nicotinic acid that overcome the flushing problems. In many cases, these have simply made the flushing reaction unpredictable. Acipimox does appear to induce less flushing, but while it retains the triglyceride-lowering action of its parent nicotinic acid, it is much less effective at lowering serum cholesterol.

CHAPTER 10
When to treat

Generally, the addition of cholesterol-lowering medication to dietary therapy has been considered cost-effective in secondary prevention (the treatment of people who already have CHD or some other clinical manifestation of atherosclerosis) and in primary intervention when the CHD risk exceeds 20% over 10 years (i.e. when more than 20 new CHD events will occur in every 100 such people over the next 10 years). Clinical trial evidence suggests that at least some people at lower levels of risk can benefit from statin therapy. However, the cost of treating people at those levels of risk would be extremely high for the tiny number who would benefit. As the cost of statin therapy decreases there may, however, be a case for decreasing the level of CHD risk at which statin treatment can be instituted cost-effectively to 15% over 10 years. Different arguments apply in the USA because the costs of healthcare are borne more directly by the patient; the same would apply to patients receiving treatment outside the state healthcare system in the UK. Thus some patients may choose to receive treatment at lower levels of risk.

Treatment should aim to reduce LDL cholesterol to below 3.0 mmol/litre (120 mg/dl) or by 30%, whichever is the lower. Some authorities argue for lower target levels, particularly in secondary prevention where they consider that 2.5 mmol/litre (100 mg/dl) or lower may be appropriate.

Identifying candidates for secondary prevention

All patients with known CHD should have careful clinical and laboratory evaluation to determine the extent of their vascular disease and to discover the factors that may have contributed to its development. With respect to the first objective, both by history and physical examination, the clinician should search for additional disease in other territories, particularly that affecting the cerebral vessels, the aorta, the renal arteries and the arteries to the lower limbs. The discovery of disease in one territory should spur new efforts to uncover it in another.

The importance of clinical diagnosis cannot be over-emphasized. About half of all myocardial infarctions occur in those with previously identifiable coronary disease and almost three-quarters of those with cardiovascular disease will die a cardiovascular death. Overall, the risk of vascular events in those with disease is at least five-fold that of those without. Thus current vascular disease is the mark of further vascular disease and vascular death in the future.

Identifying candidates for primary prevention

Currently, because the technology to recognize preclinical disease is limited and expensive, clinical assessment must be driven by discovery of the risk factors for vascular disease. These are well known (see page 41), but are unfortunately often overlooked.

The importance of identifying presymptomatic patients and individuals who will develop early and accelerated disease has led to the development of numerous guidelines from various societies around the world. They have much in common, though there are important differences of degree at which intervention is recommended. NCEP places most emphasis on the lipid profile and in particular the LDL cholesterol. The European and New Zealand guidelines place more weight on the total cardiovascular risk profile. Of the two approaches, the latter seems the more appropriate. Nevertheless, the limitations of our present approaches to recognize risk must not be overlooked. Triglycerides and HDL cholesterol measurements are not standardized and accordingly calculated LDL cholesterol is often inaccurate.

Apo B adds much and is standardized, but is not available in most clinical laboratories; the principal reason is that it is not yet included in the clinical guidelines. That is a pity because it would greatly simplify lipid evaluation for the non-specialist and add much to the diagnostic capacity for the specialist.

But even this will not solve the problem. Diabetes can be diagnosed and is an incredibly potent risk factor. But insulin resistance by routine clinical testing is not easily identified. Recently, much attention has been paid to low homocysteine levels, but again no routine laboratory evaluation is possible and in this case, there is as yet no clinical trial evidence that therapy will change outcome.

Our general rule is that the younger the patient, the greater the deviation from normal that is required to prompt preventive therapy. Unless they have markedly elevated cholesterol levels or diabetes, young women are at low risk of vascular disease. Similarly, age is the greatest risk factor for disease and we must carefully consider the merits of prevention in each of our older patients. Generally speaking, all men and women should have an assessment of risk based on a careful history and clinical evaluation to detect pre-existing vascular disease by the age of 40 years and at least every 5 years thereafter. At the same time, their cardiovascular risk factors should be measured (including cholesterol, HDL cholesterol, blood pressure and fasting glucose). In many patients, risk can be estimated using risk assessment charts, which predict the number of events that would occur in 100 people with similar risk factors over a defined time period (Figure 10.1). A computer program for calculating coronary and stroke risk can be found on the Family Heart Association website (www.familyheart.org). Additional allowance should be made for adverse family history, premature menopause, the presence of hypertriglyceridaemia, proteinuria if present, for example in diabetes, and left ventricular hypertrophy if present in hypertension; these were not included in the calculations on which the charts are based. The charts for assessment of CHD should also not be used to assess risk in patients with established vascular disease, FH, type III hyperlipo-proteinaemia, severe hypertriglyceridaemia or renal disease. Patients with Type 1 diabetes are also a special case because they tend to have relatively high levels of HDL cholesterol that does not appear to protect against CHD. In these patients, the charts can be used if the serum to HDL ratio is replaced with the serum cholesterol value alone (i.e. always making HDL cholesterol 1 mmol/litre). They can aid, but not replace, clinical judgement based on the information in this book, which is necessary in determining appropriate management.

In particularly high-risk groups, such as those with FH, type III hyperlipoproteinuria, severe hypertriglyceridaemia, renal disease and diabetes, clinical evaluation for lipid-lowering drug therapy should be made at a much earlier age than 40 years.

(a)

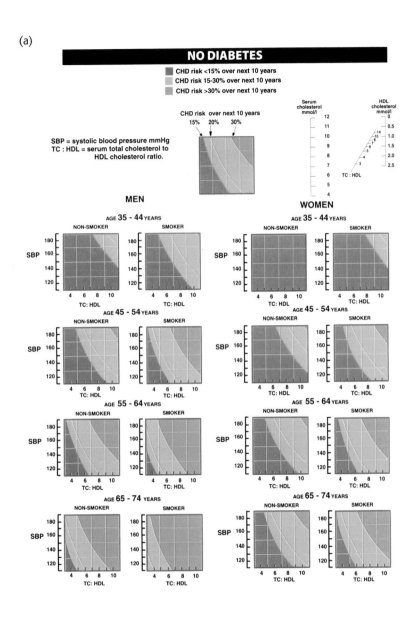

Figure 10.1 Coronary risk prediction charts for patients (a) without, and (b, facing page) with diabetes. The charts should not be used for calculating risk in people with established CHD (previous myocardial infarction and/or angina), with other significant atherosclerosis, left ventricular hypertrophy on ECG, or diabetic patients

(b)

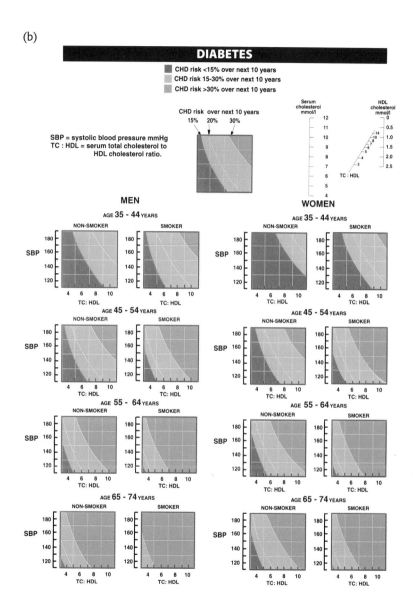

with proteinuria; these should receive lipid-lowering medication in addition to diet modification if their serum cholesterol is 5.0 mmol/litre (200 mg/dl) or above. SBP = systolic blood pressure (mmHg); TC:HDL = serum total cholesterol to HDL cholesterol ratio. Reproduced with permission from the University of Manchester, UK.

CHAPTER 11
Clinical and laboratory tests

Non-invasive diagnostic methods for asymptomatic atherosclerosis

These need to be simple, inexpensive and widely available. The electro-cardiogram fulfils all of these criteria and although it is only rarely helpful in the asymptomatic patient, the test should not be neglected. Bruits in peripheral vessels should be examined with Doppler ultrasound. Treadmill exercise tests are often essential to diagnose chest pain accurately and to determine the ischaemic threshold. Echocardiography is not a screening tool to recognize coronary disease, and neither are the more sophisticated stress tests, such as treadmill stress testing, stress echocardiography or radionuclide stress imaging.

Biochemical laboratory tests

Methodological sources of variability. Accuracy describes how closely the results from the particular technique being used in a specific laboratory relate to the results obtained using the accepted reference (or best) method for that variable. That is, how close is the answer in your laboratory to the right answer? All other things being equal, any deviation from the reference method should be systematic. Lack of accuracy or 'bias' makes comparison of results difficult (if not impossible), and therefore the application of guidelines difficult (if not impossible).

Precision quantitates the difference in repeated measures of the same sample and is expressed as the coefficient of variation (the standard deviation of the repeated measures divided by their average). That is, how variable would the results from the laboratory be if the same sample were measured repeatedly?

Precision and accuracy should each be less than 3%. Even within these limits, there can be considerable variance in laboratory reports for the same sample, which is why it is recommended to sample more than once before categorizing lipid levels.

Another criterion to consider is standardization. A test is said to be standardized when all methods that have been approved for routine clinical use yield the same value, because all have been related to an accepted reference. Standardized tests allow results from the same patient, but from different laboratories, to be compared.

Unfortunately, while considerable progress has been made in improving clinical lipid testing, important limitations remain. Only total cholesterol and apo B and apo A1 meet all the requirements.

Biological sources of variability are multiple and can be separated into physiological, behavioural and clinical sources of variability.

Age, gender and diet are important modifiers of plasma lipid levels (see pages 19 and 26). Clinical factors also need to be taken into account. For example, lipid levels change abruptly and markedly with many illnesses (e.g. myocardial infarction) and operations (e.g. coronary artery bypass surgery) making accurate diagnosis in the acute setting difficult, if not impossible. Serum cholesterol measured within 24 hours of the onset of chest pain in patients with acute myocardial infarction or coronary insufficiency can be a guide to how high the cholesterol was before the acute event. However, it should never be concluded that a level of below 5.0 mmol/litre (200 mg/dl) measured under these circumstances means that statin therapy is unnecessary. In all patients, subsequent levels should be obtained. Certain medications including steroid sex hormones can also affect lipid levels (see Chapter 7).

Total cholesterol. Almost all clinical laboratories now use enzymatic techniques to measure cholesterol and the measurement is rapid, accurate and easily automated. Non-fasting samples can be used. An abnormally high total cholesterol can occasionally be due to either markedly increased HDL cholesterol or chylomicrons. With the latter, depending on the level of triglycerides, the risk of pancreatitis may be augmented.

The virtues of total cholesterol measurement are its simplicity and reliability. The drawbacks are that, with the exception of a small minority with markedly high values, there is little difference between the cholesterol levels of those with and those without coronary disease. Moreover, mild or moderate elevation in LDL cholesterol with concomitant reduction in HDL cholesterol may result in a normal total cholesterol value.

Triglycerides. Enzymatic methods are also the most commonly used means to measure plasma triglycerides. However, these methods are less precise, less accurate and not standardized. Furthermore, as plasma triglycerides rise markedly after a meal due to the entry into plasma of dietary fatty acids such as chylomicron triglycerides, standard practice calls for fasting samples so that generally VLDL triglycerides only will be measured. This imposes considerable difficulty for the patient and considerable uncertainty for the laboratory. However, many patients with coronary disease have impaired chylomicron clearance from plasma after meals and the increased remnants may contribute to their risk of vascular disease. This feature is difficult to assess in clinical practice if only fasting samples are taken. However, such patients frequently also have an elevated apo B.

LDL cholesterol has become the benchmark laboratory test on which most therapeutic decisions are based. It has many strengths and its value is supported by the epidemiological and therapeutic data gathered over considerable time. Another important advantage is that it is now familiar to many physicians the world over. But it has important limitations and these should not be overlooked.

First, in most laboratories, it is a calculated value rather than a direct measurement. The usual formulae used are:

$$[\text{LDL cholesterol}] = [\text{total cholesterol}] - \left([\text{HDL cholesterol}] + \frac{[\text{triglycerides}]}{2.2}\right)$$

if all concentrations are in mmol/litre;

$$[\text{LDL cholesterol}] = [\text{total cholesterol}] - \left([\text{HDL cholesterol}] + \frac{[\text{triglycerides}]}{5}\right)$$

if all concentrations are in mg/dl. Therefore, all the inaccuracies in each test come into play.

Second, it is not standardized and therefore values gained using one method are not necessarily the same as those gained using another, making the application of guidelines somewhat imprecise.

Third, just as with total cholesterol, there is so much overlap in the values of LDL cholesterol between those with and those without coronary disease, unless levels are markedly elevated, it is of little use. This point is crucial. In societies with high rates of CHD, most patients with coronary disease do not have levels of LDL cholesterol elevated above those of the general population. One of the most extensive studies in North America demonstrated that only 23% of patients with coronary disease had a total cholesterol level above 6.2 mmol/litre (240 mg/dl). This does not mean that LDL particle number is not commonly elevated in patients with coronary disease, even though LDL cholesterol is only average for the population as a whole.

Fourth, fasting samples are required (because triglyceride values are required in the formula) with all the attendant disadvantages this poses.

HDL cholesterol is measured in most clinical laboratories by first precipitating the apo B-containing lipoproteins (VLDL, IDL and LDL) and then measuring cholesterol in the supernatant. There is considerable epidemiological evidence demonstrating that the risk of coronary disease is inversely related to the level of HDL cholesterol. The measurement also has considerable limitations. It is not standardized, and accuracy is particularly critical as there are, in general, only small differences between normal and abnormal levels. Also, it is not clear how a low HDL cholesterol increases the risk of disease. This limitation matters because a low HDL cholesterol frequently coexists with other abnormalities such as a high triglyceride or high apo B value. Furthermore, there is no pharmacological therapy currently available that increases HDL cholesterol only, thus no clinical trials have focused on this effect in isolation.

Total serum cholesterol:HDL cholesterol. This ratio may provide a better approach; it is, for example, the method used in the charts in Figure 10.1 (see pages 98–99) and includes the risk embodied in LDL cholesterol. There is a wealth of epidemiological data relating to it and it is therapeutically modifiable by drugs such as statins, albeit because of their effects on LDL cholesterol rather than HDL cholesterol. The ratio also contains in the HDL cholesterol value much of the prognostic information contained in triglyceride values, because these are strongly inversely correlated to HDL. It may also therefore have an advantage over serum non-HDL cholesterol (serum cholesterol – HDL cholesterol) values, which have also been proposed as overcoming some of the difficulties posed by indirect estimation of LDL cholesterol.

Apo B. Each VLDL particle secreted by the liver contains one molecule of apo B_{100}, which stays with the particle for its biological life. Thus the metabolic products of VLDL, IDL and LDL also contain one molecule of apo B_{100}. Consequently, measuring the plasma apo B gives an exact measure of the total number of atherogenic VLDL, IDL and LDL particles in plasma. Of these, more than 90% are LDL. Thus plasma apo B acts as a close surrogate for LDL particle number. As discussed earlier, LDL particles are heterogeneous in composition and LDL cholesterol does not correspond to the number of LDL particles. This is important because in CHD, cholesteryl ester-depleted, smaller, denser LDL are so common. Unless apo B is measured, an elevation in LDL particle number will not always be recognized.

Standardized, automated, accurate and precise methods of measuring plasma apo B have only recently become available. These principally measure apo B_{100} contained in VLDL, IDL and LDL. In chylomicrons, even in the peak postprandial hyperlipidaemic state, there are few chylomicron apo B_{48} particles. Thus fasting samples are not necessary to measure and interpret plasma apo B_{100}. The level of plasma apo B has been prospectively shown to relate to the risk of CHD and also, interestingly, to the risk of developing Type 2 diabetes.

Apo AI, one of the major apolipoproteins in HDL, can also be accurately and precisely measured using standardized assays. There is an inverse correlation with risk, as there is with HDL cholesterol. However, there appears to be no prognostic information additional to that available from HDL cholesterol and indeed it may be less informative.

Lp(a). For now, Lp(a) can only be measured in a few laboratories. Considerable work remains to be done in standardizing the assay before it could be broadly introduced into clinical practice (see page 105).

CHAPTER 12
Future trends

Clinical measurements

Apo B. Given that apo B measurement has been standardized and it is neither difficult nor expensive to perform, it should be possible to overcome the arguments against its introduction as a routine test. On the other hand, there seems little argument for measuring apo AI, the major apolipoprotein in HDL, because HDL cholesterol seems to be more informative.

Small, dense LDL increases the risk of vascular disease. As increased LDL particle number and small, dense LDL often coexist, it has been difficult to be sure of the degree of risk conferred by the small, dense LDL. However, the Quebec Cardiovascular Study has demonstrated that an elevated apo B doubles the risk of coronary disease and small, dense LDL increases the risk six-fold. There are no routine methods currently available for the detection of small, dense LDL. However, a plasma triglyceride level over 1.5 mmol/litre should raise suspicion of the presence of small, dense LDL.

Lp(a) is present in serum, and shows considerable interindividual variation. Its level is related to CHD and stroke risk. It is greatly increased in patients with any type of renal disease and in many patients with FH. Lp(a) measurement is not currently available for routine patient evaluation. It may, however, assume greater importance if a safe and effective therapeutic approach to lowering Lp(a) appears and is shown to decrease the incidence of vascular disease. The measurement of Lp(a) will have to be improved as the marked variations in its composition and molecular weight make comparison amongst individuals more difficult than is usually recognized.

Plasma homocysteine. Much interest has been generated by recent studies linking increased risk of vascular disease to increased plasma homocysteine levels. However, until clinical trial evidence and its routine measurement become available, it will be impossible to incorporate homocysteine into routine clinical practice. Physicians will have to continue to use their clinical judgement as to whether folate supplementation should be given to patients with vascular disease.

Plasma fibrinogen and plasminogen activator inhibitor increases have also been linked to increased risk. More information is needed on how much their measurement adds to risk assessment , particularly after other risk factors are included in the evaluation. Overall, however, any final strategy of risk assessment will ideally include a thorough evaluation of a range of prothrombogenic factors.

New methods to diagnose presymptomatic vascular disease

This is the area in which the greatest progress should be made. Methods are needed to identify early non-occlusive vascular disease. At the moment, carotid ultrasound is helpful at least with respect to moderate lesions. Unfortunately, at present, the technique is too operator-dependent and too expensive to be widely available. At least the proximal portions of the coronary arteries can be visualized by transoesophageal echocardiography, but this will never be a practical general screening method. Ultrafast computed tomography can detect coronary calcification and this relates at least in a general way to the extent of coronary disease. The method is non-invasive but may not be sufficiently selective to be of practical value. Magnetic resonance imaging of the coronary arteries holds great promise, but expense may unfortunately limit its widespread use.

Clinical trials

The first-generation clinical trials of primary and secondary prevention showed that LDL lowering reduced clinical events without significant side-effects. But they do not define the therapeutic targets. There are other important objectives for clinical trials. Are triglyceride-lowering agents effective and if so what is the mechanism responsible? Does combination therapy add to clinical benefit? We must also acknowledge that we lack definitive knowledge about the value of lipid-lowering therapy in critical subgroups. At least numerically, people with diabetes may make up the largest group. The initial trials suggest substantial benefit from LDL lowering. However, the lipid profiles of the diabetics in these trials is not typically encountered and subgroup analyses do not substitute for a primary test of the hypothesis.

All in all, there is much still to be learnt about hyperlipidaemia and its role in disease prevention. However, there is a great deal that still needs to be done in clinical practice to take full advantage of what is already known. An important and realisable objective for the immediate future is to implement fully our existing knowledge of the treatment of hyperlipidaemia.

Key references

LIPIDS AND LIPOPROTEINS

Cahill GF. Starvation in man. *N Engl J Med* 1970;282:668–75.

Durrington PN. Lipids and their metabolism. In: *Hyperlipidaemia, Diagnosis and Management*. 2nd edn. Oxford: Butterworth Heinemann, 1995:4–24.

Durrington PN. Lipoproteins and their metabolism. In: *Hyperlipidaemia, Diagnosis and Management*. 2nd edn. Oxford: Butterworth Heinemann, 1995:25–71.

Gibons GF, Mitropoulos K, Myant NB. *Biochemistry of Cholesterol*. 4th edn. Amsterdam: Elsevier, 1982.

Gurr MI, James AT. *Lipid Biochemistry: an Introduction*. London: Chapman and Hall, 1991.

Packard CJ, Shepherd J. Physiology of the lipoprotein transport system: an overview of lipoprotein metabolism. In: Betteridge DJ *et al.*, eds. *Lipoproteins in Health and Disease*. London: Arnold, 1999:17–30.

EPIDEMIOLOGY AND PATHOPHYSIOLOGY

Charlton J, Murphy M, Khaw K *et al.* Cardiovascular diseases. In: Charlton J *et al.*, eds. *The Health of Adult Britain 1841–1994*. Vol. 2. London: The Stationery Office, 1997:60–81.

Charlton J, Quaife K. Trends in diet 1841–1994. In: Charlton J *et al.*, eds. *The Health of Adult Britain 1841–1994*. Vol. 1. London: The Stationery Office, 1997:93–113.

Gordon DJ. Epidemiology of lipoproteins. In: Betteridge DJ *et al.*, eds. *Lipoproteins in Health and Disease*. London: Arnold, 1999:587–95.

Law MR, Wald NJ, Thompson SG. By how much and how quickly does reduction in serum cholesterol concentration lower risk of ischaemic heart disease? *BMJ* 1994;308:367–72.

Ross R. The pathogenesis of atherosclerosis: a perspective for the 1990s. *Nature* 1993;362:801–9.

Steinberg D. Low density lipoprotein oxidation and its pathobiological significance. *J Biol Chem* 1997; 272:20963–6.

FAMILIAL (MONOGENIC) HYPERCHOLESTEROLAEMIA

Durrington PN. Familial hypercholesterolaemia. In: *Hyperlipidaemia, Diagnosis and Management*. Oxford: Butterworth Heinemann, 1995:108–39.

Goldstein JL, Hobbs HH, Brown MS. Familial hypercholesterolaemia. In: Scriver CR *et al.*, eds. *The Metabolic and Molecular Bases of Inherited Disease*. Vol. 2. 7th edn. New York: McGraw Hill, 1995:1981–2030.

POLYGENIC AND FAMILIAL COMBINED HYPERLIPIDAEMIAS

Durrington P. Lipid and lipoprotein disorders. In: Weatherall DJ *et al.*, eds. *Oxford Textbook of Medicine*. Vol. 2. 3rd edn. Oxford: Oxford University Press, 1996:1399–415.

Jarvik GP, Austin MA, Brunzell JD. Familial combined hyperlipidaemia. In: Betteridge DJ *et al.*, eds. *Lipoproteins in Health and Disease*. London: Arnold, 1999:693–9.

Sniderman AD, Pedersen T, Kjekshus J. Putting low-density lipoproteins at center stage in atherogenesis. *Am J Cardiol* 1997;79:64–7.

HYPERTRIGLYCERIDAEMIA

Brunzell JD. Familial lipoprotein lipase deficiency and other causes of chylomicronemia syndrome. In: Scriver CR *et al.*, eds. *The Metabolic and Molecular Bases of Inherited Disease*. Vol. 2. 7th edn. New York: McGraw Hill, 1995:1913–32.

Durrington PN. Hypertriglyceridaemia. In: *Hyperlipidaemia, Diagnosis and Management*. 2nd edn. Oxford: Butterworth Heinemann, 1995:190–214.

Durrington PN. Triglycerides are more important than epidemiology has suggested. *Atherosclerosis* 1998;141(Suppl 1):S57–62.

TYPE III HYPERLIPOPROTEINAEMIA

Mahley RW, Rall SC. Type III hyperlipoproteinemia (dysbetalipoproteinemia): the role of apolipoprotein E in normal and abnormal lipoprotein metabolism. In: Scriver CR *et al.*, eds. *Metabolic and Molecular Bases of Inherited Disease*. New York: McGraw Hill, 1995:1953–80.

National Institute on Ageing. The Alzheimer's Association Working Group. Apolipoprotein E genotyping in Alzheimer's disease. *Lancet* 1996;347:1091–5.

SECONDARY HYPERLIPIDAEMIA

Baraona E, Lieber CS. Alcohol. In: Betteridge DJ *et al.*, eds. *Lipoproteins in Health and Disease*. London: Arnold, 1999:1011–36.

Durrington PN. Secondary hyperlipidaemia. In: *Hyperlipidaemia, Diagnosis and Management*. Oxford: Butterworth Heinemann, 1995:291–360.

Edwards CM, Stacpoole PW. Rare secondary dyslipidaemias. In: Betteridge DJ *et al.*, eds. *Lipoproteins in Health and Disease*. London: Arnold, 1999:1069–98.

Kissebah AH, Krakower GR. Endocrine disorders. In: Betteridge DJ *et al.*, eds. *Lipoproteins in Health and Disease*. London: Arnold, 1999:931–41.

Lean MEJ. Obesity and eating disorders. In: Betteridge DJ *et al.*, eds. *Lipoproteins in Health and Disease*. London: Arnold, 1999:881–95.

Miller JP. Liver disease. In: Betteridge DJ *et al.*, eds. *Lipoproteins in Health and Disease*. London: Arnold, 1999: 985–1009.

Muller-Wieland D, Krone W. Drug-induced effects. In: Betteridge DJ *et al.*, eds. *Lipoproteins in Health and Disease*. London: Arnold, 1999:1037–48.

Short CD, Durrington PN. Renal disorders. In: Betteridge DJ *et al.*, eds. *Lipoproteins in Health and Disease*. London: Arnold, 1999:943–66.

DIETARY TREATMENT

Durrington PN. Diet. In: *Hyperlipidaemia, Diagnosis and Management*. Oxford: Butterworth Heinemann, 1995:225–57.

Grundy SM. Dietary therapy of hyperlipidaemia. *Baillieres Clin Endocrinol Metab* 1987;1:667–98.

DRUG TREATMENT

Ballantyne CM, Herd JA, Dunn JK *et al.* Effects of lipid-lowering therapy on progression of coronary and carotid artery disease. *Curr Opin Lipidol* 1997;8:354–61.

Downs JR, Clearfield M, Weis S *et al.* Primary prevention of acute coronary events with lovastatin in men and women with average cholesterol levels. Results of AFACPS/TexCAPS. *JAMA* 1998;279: 1615–22.

Rubins HB, Rubins SJ, Collins D *et al.* Gemfibrozil for the secondary prevention of coronary heart disease in men with low levels of high-density lipoprotein cholesterol. *N Engl J Med* 1999; 341:410–18.

Sacks FM, Pfeffer MA, Moye LA *et al.* The effect of pravastatin on coronary events after myocardial infarction in patients with average cholesterol levels. *N Engl J Med* 1996;335:1001–9.

Scandinavian Simvastatin Survival Study Group. Randomised trial of cholesterol lowering in 4444 patients with coronary heart disease; the Scandinavian Survival Study. *Lancet* 1994;344:1383–9.

Shepherd J, Cobbe SM, Ford I *et al.*, for the West of Scotland Coronary Prevention Study Group. Prevention of coronary heart disease with pravastatin in men with hypercholesterolaemia. *N Engl J Med* 1995;333:1301–7.

The Long-Term Intervention with Pravastatin in Ischaemic Heart Disease (LIPID) Study Group. Prevention of cardiovascular events and death with pravastatin in patients with coronary heart disease and a broad range of initial cholesterol levels. *N Engl J Med* 1998;339:1349–57.

WHEN TO TREAT

Durrington PN, Prais H, Bhatnagar D *et al.* Indications for the cholesterol-lowering medication: comparison of risk-assessment methods. *Lancet* 1999;353:278–81.

NCEP (National Cholesterol Education Program) Guidelines of the Second Adult Treatment Panel (ATPII). *JAMA* 1993;267:3015–23.

Sniderman AD. Counterpoint. To measure apo B or not to: a critique of modern medical decision-making. *Clin Chem* 1997;43:1310–14.

Wood D, Durrington PN, Poulter N *et al.* Joint British Recommendations on prevention of coronary heart disease in clinical practice. *Heart* 1998;80 (Suppl 2): S1–29.

CLINICAL AND LABORATORY TESTS

Rifai N, Warnick GR, Dominiczak MH, eds. *Handbook of Lipoprotein Testing.* Washington: American Association for Clinical Chemistry Press, 1997.

FUTURE TRENDS

Suckling K, Fears R. Future developments in drug therapy. In: Betteridge DJ *et al.*, eds. *Lipoproteins in Health and Disease.* London: Arnold, 1999:1267–77.

Index

Other titles available in the *Fast Facts* series

Asthma
by Stephen T Holgate and Romain A Pauwels

Allergic Rhinitis
by Niels Mygind and Glenis K Scadding

Benign Prostatic Hyperplasia (third edition)
by Roger S Kirby and John D McConnell

Coeliac Disease
by Geoffrey Holmes and Carlo Catassi

Contraception
by Anna Glasier and Beverly Winikoff

Diseases of the Testis
by Timothy J Christmas, Michael D Dinneen and Larry Lipshultz

Dyspepsia
by Michael J Lancaster Smith and Kenneth L Koch

Endometriosis
by Hossam Abdalla and Botros Rizk

Epilepsy
by Martin J Brodie and Steven C Schachter

Headaches
by Richard Peatfield and J Keith Campbell

Hyperlipidaemia
by Paul Durrington and Allan Sniderman

Irritable Bowel Syndrome
by Kenneth W Heaton and W Grant Thompson

Menopause
by David H Barlow and Barry G Wren

Stress and Strain
by Cary L Cooper and James Campbell Quick

Urinary Continence
by Julian Shah and Gary Leach

To order, please contact:

Health Press Limited
Elizabeth House, Queen Street,
Abingdon, Oxford OX14 3JR, UK
Tel: +44 (0)1235 523233
Fax: +44 (0)1235 523238
Email: post@healthpress.co.uk

Or visit our website:
www.healthpress.co.uk

Health Press
medical publishing at its best

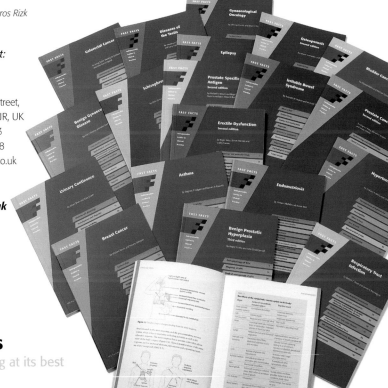